T0342314

Comprehensive Occlusal Concepts in Clinical Practice

Comprehensive Occlusal Concepts in Clinical Practice

Irwin M. Becker, DDS

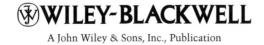

A John Wiley & Sons, Inc., Publication

This edition first published 2011 © 2011 by Blackwell Publishing, Ltd.

Blackwell Publishing was acquired by John Wiley & Sons in February 2007. Blackwell's publishing program has been merged with Wiley's global Scientific, Technical and Medical business to form Wiley-Blackwell.

Registered office: John Wiley & Sons Ltd, The Atrium, Southern Gate, Chichester, West Sussex, PO19 8SQ, UK

Editorial offices: 2121 State Avenue, Ames, Iowa 50014-8300, USA
9600 Garsington Road, Oxford, OX4 2DQ, UK

For details of our global editorial offices, for customer services and for information about how to apply for permission to reuse the copyright material in this book please see our website at www.wiley.com/wiley-blackwell.

Library of Congress Cataloging-in-Publication Data

Comprehensive occlusal concepts in clinical practice / [edited by] Irwin M. Becker.
      p. ; cm.
   Includes bibliographical references and index.
   ISBN 978-0-8138-0584-9 (pbk. : alk. paper) 1. Malocclusion. I. Becker, Irwin, 1943-
   [DNLM: 1. Malocclusion–therapy.   2. Malocclusion–physiopathology. WU 440]
   RK523.C66 2011
   617.6'43–dc22
                              2010028088

A catalogue record for this book is available from the British Library.

This book is published in the following electronic formats: eBook 9780470958643; ePub 9780470958650

Set in 9.5/12 pt Palatino by Toppan Best-set Premedia Limited

Disclaimer

1   2011

Contents

Preface

In order to encapsulate and organize the body of occlusal knowledge that I have been learning, attempting to apply for the benefit of my patients, and teaching over the past 40 years, I committed to write this text. I hope it will help those who struggle to understand the seemingly complex subject of dental occlusion. I still meet dentists from all over the world who tell me that the subject remains confusing and is somewhat of an illusion. Many articles that I read question the role of occlusion in everyday dentistry. There are research articles that attempt to demonstrate evidence that occlusion simply doesn't matter. Lastly, some of the most talented and educated clinicians still make presentations of beautiful maxillary ceramic restorations that do not come close to matching their opposing mandibular incisal edges.

Because these examples are still common and yet puzzling to those of us who have come to appreciate the clinical importance of the role of occlusion, this text is really dedicated to all the giants of our profession who have influenced and motivated many of us to seek out the clinical significance of this topic. In reality, this is my way of thanking those who have taught and challenged me and caused me to question what I thought I understood about how the masticatory system functions. These same mentors taught me and many others that the success of our profession is dependent on the classical process of examination, diagnosis, reasonable verification of diagnosis, and appropriate treatment planning.

In dental school I had several professors who made significant impact on my thinking about occlusion and comprehensive care. Most notable was Dr. Richard Wilson of Maynard and Wilson fame relative to modern understanding of biologic width. I had the privilege to work closely with Dr. Marvin Reynolds, who taught me the basics of gnathology and helped me with my first occlusal reconstruction. My journey toward comprehensive care continued with my studies and work in the Prosthodontic Residency Program at Boston University. My greatest influences came from Drs. Gerry Kramer, Ron Nevins, Don Mori, Leo Talkov, and Howard Skurow. When I began my practice in Miami, my journey benefited from giants in restorative dentistry such as Dr. Peter Dawson and Dr. Robert Kaplan, who really began the process of organizing the concepts of occlusion. Of course, it was also at this time that I had the opportunity to learn from Dr. L. D. Pankey. I would be remiss to not mention the influence Dr. Lloyd Miller had on me in developing the thoughts of combining function and esthetics as one comprehensive subject.

However, I have come to understand that my raging passion for comprehensive, optimal care and my insatiable search for occlusal truth actually began with a dental appointment when I was 16 years old. The dentist who performed a comprehensive examination and subsequently restored my lower right first molar with a gold onlay sparked a lifelong quest to understand how and why his restoration has been successful for over 50 years. You see, Dr. David Seitlin not only placed an exquisite restoration, he also equilibrated my bite at that time. And perhaps most important, the manner in which he did the co-discovery led to an immediate change in my appreciation of dentistry, Dr. Seitlin's style practice, and my understanding of my own dental condition. Although I didn't understand at that time why he was doing certain things such as utilizing a face bow registration, the way he did things comprehensively changed my viewpoint of dentistry, and I began to consider a career in dentistry. I will be forever grateful for his manner of treating patients.

My goal for this text is to appropriately represent the knowledge base that has been shared with me over these many decades. I hope the knowledge I have will never get in the way of new learning and new methods of application. Today, I am working hard to blend the newest digital technologies with classical comprehensive approaches to restorative dentistry in order to ensure longevity, comfort, predictability, function, and natural beauty.

I would not have been able to be in the position to write this text if it were not for the love and support of my wife of 46 years. Susie has always realized what my dedication to optimal dentistry has meant to me, and her personal sacrifices and encouragement have made it possible for me to have a wonderful and fulfilling career in practicing and teaching the subjects that I hold most precious.

Acknowledgement goes to my personal editor, Deb Bush, who spent countless hours turning my thoughts into readable text material. Her expertise as not only an editor but someone who understands the goals of comprehensive care as well as any dentist I have ever been associated with surely makes a significant difference in the clarity of this text. All of my associates at the Pankey Institute have taught me and shared with me their own learning journey, so much so that I am convinced that no one has learned more studying there than me. And clearly all my students who have challenged my beliefs and asked the right questions surely taught me the most. I lastly recognize the input of my son, Daren Becker, whose comments over this text helped make it more understandable and useful as a representative of my years of teaching.

Contributors

Irwin M. Becker, DDS
Chairman of the Department of Education
The Pankey Institute for Advanced Dental Education
1 Crandon Boulevard
Key Biscayne, FL 33142

Herbert E. Blumenthal, DDS
Visiting Faculty, The Pankey Institute, Key Biscayne, FL
Private Practice, Cordova, TN
280 German Oak Drive
Cordova, TN 38018

Henry A. Gremillion, DDS, MAGD
Professor, Department of Orthodontics
Dean, Louisiana State University Health Sciences Center School
of Dentistry
LSU School of Dentistry
1100 Florida Avenue
New Orleans, LA 70119

Stephen K. Harrel, DDS
Professor of Periodontology, Baylor College of Dentistry, Dallas, TX
Private Practice, Dallas, TX
10246 Midway Road, #101
Dallas, Texas 75229

Martha E. Nunn, DDS, PhD
Director, Center for Oral Health Research
Associate Professor, Periodontics
School of Dentistry
Creighton University
2500 California Plaza
Omaha, NE 68178

Matthew R. Roberts, CDT
Founder of CRM Dental Laboratory and Team Aesthetics Seminars
Team Aesthetics
185 South Capital Ave.
Idaho Falls, ID 83402

Roger A. Solow, DDS
Visiting Faculty, The Pankey Institute, Key Biscayne, FL
Private Practice, Mill Valley, CA
655 Redwood Highway #251
Mill Valley, CA, 94941

Christopher J. Spencer, DDS
Clinical Assistant Professor Department of Restorative Dental Sciences
Department of Comprehensive Dentistry
University of Florida College of Dentistry
1600 SW Archer Road
Gainesville, FL 32610

Comprehensive Occlusal Concepts in Clinical Practice

Introduction to Occlusal Disease and Rationale for Occlusal Therapy

Irwin M. Becker, DDS

To understand the reasoning and general purpose of entering into any therapy that may change or modify a patient's occlusal scheme, it is important to first realize that most signs and symptoms of occlusal causation occur mainly in individuals who demonstrate some degree of *parafunctional activity*. That is to say, a sign such as attrition rarely occurs from normal mastication (Belser and Hannam, 1985; MacDonald and Hannam, 1984; Moss et al., 1987; Silvestri, Cohen, and Connolly, 1980).

INTRODUCTORY DISCUSSION OF PARAFUNCTIONAL WEAR

Almost no one spends sufficient time with their teeth in contact during normal chewing function to cause observable wear patterns. These common wear patterns come from those times of clenching and or bruxing during either nocturnal or diurnal time frames. The potential etiologies of these activities will be discussed in chapter 2.

Of course, there are exceptions to the statement that parafunctional habits are the overriding, most common cause of signs and symptoms of occlusal disease. Conditions such as iatrogenic changes or dual bites, where a patient holds his or her teeth in a position other than some acquired closing pattern, could be considered additional causes of signs of occlusal disease (Attanasio, 1991; Kampe, 1987).

It is also essential for the modern dental clinician to understand that there exists a clear clinical ability to reduce muscle activity during these parafunctionally destructive times, but no clear evidence exists that the clinician can reduce or stop the actual parafunctional habits. The total body of evidence indicates that by providing a physiologic occlusion, a therapist can realistically reduce the muscle activity during bruxing and clenching. The therapist can greatly reduce the results of a destructive habit, realizing that the habit itself remains; only the muscle activity is reduced (Ash, 2006; Baba, 1991; Geering, 1974).

Most of this text will further explain this basic concept and help the reader develop understanding and learn multiple techniques proven to achieve the physiologic occlusion mentioned above. It is necessary first to master the ability to recognize and then categorize all the potential signs and symptoms that make up any given disease (Lytle, 1990, 2001a, 2001b). As in all scientific methodologies utilized in medical and dental practices, there are accepted protocols. These protocols are summarized by detailed examination, varying diagnostic procedures, and treatment planning opportunities when and where appropriate.

RATIONALE FOR COMPREHENSIVE OCCLUSAL EXAMINATION

Obviously, dental examinations must be comprehensive and thorough. But they must be more than a detailed collection of data. The examination is usually performed after any emergencies or other compelling issues have been addressed. Once the patient's perceived chief complaints or concerns have been addressed, the doctor-patient relationship is more likely to lead to an engaged patient ready to interact with the dentist during the comprehensive clinical examination.

It should be mentioned at this time that there is evidence that pain is not a reliable indicator of the presence of occlusal disease. Epidemiological studies have consistently shown that in large groups of subjects, those with malocclusion have no more pain than those with more ideal occlusal schemes (Kampe, Hannerz, Strom, 1991; Okeson, 1981; Wadhwa and Kapila, 2008). Many clinicians have observed this phenomenon in their own practices, sometimes observing patients with horrible malocclusions who have almost no symptoms. They present with no complaints of pain or discomfort. When these same patients also have no signs, it is then apparent that they spend very little time in parafunctional activity. This is further rationale for a comprehensive occlusal examination to carefully list any present signs and symptoms, as they are a strong indicator of the history of what has taken place on the dentition.

Table 1.1. Categories of parafunctional activity.

TYPE 1:	No evidence of wear, mobility, tooth migration, muscle
Almost No Parafunction	soreness, fractures, cracks, craze lines, or abfractive lesions
TYPE 2:	Evidence of slight wear, mobility, tooth migration, muscle
Moderate Parafunction	soreness, fractures, cracks, craze lines, or abfractive lesions
TYPE 3:	Evidence of excessive wear, mobility, tooth migration, muscle
Destructive Parafunction	soreness, fractures, cracks, craze lines, or abfractive lesions

CATEGORIES OF PARAFUNCTIONAL ACTIVITY

After a comprehensive occlusal examination, the clinician should be able to classify a given patient in one of the three categories outlined in table 1.1 (Lytle 1990, 2001a, 2001b).

ENGAGING THE PATIENT IN THE COMPREHENSIVE OCCLUSAL EXAM

It must be stated clearly now that it cannot be simply left up to the patient to say whether he or she has a parafunctional habit or not. Consistently, the literature suggests that these activities occur either during sleep or at times of stress (Campillo et al., 2008; Glaros et al., 2000; Kevij, Mehulic, and Dundjer, 2007; Wood, 1987). Either way, the patient is generally not aware of these occurrences. It can become quite instructive and helpful for patients to discover the destructive effects of their own habits as the process of co-discovery occurs.

If the clinician asks open-ended questions for the patient to ponder as the patient is shown the results of heretofore-unrealized habits, the patient may discover the destructive effects during the interactive exam process or realize the relationship after the exam. Commonly, patients realize they have been "chewing up their own dentition." This discovery helps the patient accept recommended phase I treatment such as occlusal splint therapy.

RATIONALE FOR OCCLUSAL THERAPY

The various signs that are detected during a routine yet thorough occlusal exam are usually repeatable and measurable, and they are the best indicators of occlusal disease. It is appropriate for the comprehensive dentist to perform this type of examination prior to determining the category of parafunction present in the patient's history and prior to treatment planning. The dentist only has a scientific basis for providing definitive occlusal therapy when the patient has clinical signs of occlusal disease (Clark et al.,

1999; Machado et al., 2007; Okamoto et al., 2000; Ratcliff, Becker, and Quinn, 2001; Speck, 1988).

Unless there exists a need to change the acquired occlusion because of orthodontic or restorative requirements, there is little literature-based support for therapies such as occlusal equilibration. Even when signs and symptoms do exist, it is important for the clinician to prove that these signs are directly related to occlusal factors. Only if there is evidence of occlusal instability or parafunction should the clinician attempt to modify the occlusion. When there is no evidence, the clinician should leave the patient with his or her wonderfully adapted and acquired occlusal scheme.

Some discussion is needed at this time about the literature involved with noncarious cervical lesions (Braem, Lambrecht, and Vanherle, 1982; Dejak, Mlotkowski, and Romanowicz, 2005; Grippo, 1991; Grippo and Simring, 1995; Kuroe et al., 2001; Lee and Eakle, 1996; Madani and Ahmadian-Yazdi, 2005; Pegoraro et al., 2005; Pintado et al., 2000; Spranger, 1995; Winter and Allen, 2005). It is common for clinicians to assume that these wedge-shaped lesions have an occlusal traumatic etiology. Even though there exists some conflicting literature, it has yet to be scientifically proven that abfraction solely occurs as a result of occlusal trauma. More likely, it is a result of a multifactorial phenomenon of trauma, lack of buccal bone, prominence of the root, and some tooth brushing and tooth paste abuse. The clinician has little choice but to include all of these possibilities in thinking about what to do with a dentition that has some abfractive lesions. When these lesions are present and there is evidence of occlusal trauma, the clinician should remove occlusal trauma as one of the possible etiologic factors.

If root prominence exists, orthodontics could be helpful. There may be a rationale for gingival grafting to protect the root with attached gingival. This is just one example of the complexity and sophistication needed to accurately define the cause and effect of many so-called multifactorial conditions in dentistry and medicine.

THE COMPREHENSIVE OCCCLUSAL EXAMINATION

A comprehensive occlusal examination must include but not necessarily be limited to the following components:

- Occlusal analysis (described below)
- Muscle palpation (described in chapter 6)
- Range of motion (described below)
- Joint sounds (described below)
- Joint palpation (described below)
- Articulated study casts (described below)
- CR (centric relation) analysis (described below)
- Digital imaging (described below)

Occlusal Analysis

Marking the teeth with appropriate ribbons after drying them with tissue paper folded on a Miller Forceps allows the clinician to identify what parts of the teeth touch during arc of closure as well as excursive movements. These markings indicate which occlusal surfaces can touch during patient instruction but not necessarily what the patient actually does during parafunctional movements. The clinician must look for actual evidence during the rest of the exam to correlate these markings with recordable signs such as wear or mobility. This process can be another learning moment for the patient, when both the patient and the dentist see and feel these contacts. The patient can feel them by rubbing the teeth together, and the clinician can feel them by placing slight pressure on the tooth in question with a finger while the patient rubs the teeth together.

Two different-colored ribbons (red and black) should be utilized to differentiate closure markings from excursive markings. Excursive movements are marked first with red, and then closure movements are marked with black. This is further described in chapter 10, which covers the details of equilibration. It will become easy for the clinician to identify working, balancing, and protrusive markings and understand the potential damaging effects from these excursive interferences.

The mechanism of micro trauma during parafunctional repetition of these contacts, both on the teeth and joint apparatus, is discussed in chapter 10. Suffice it to say at this time that the major causes of joint deterioration occur as a result of external trauma (a blow to the face or jaw) and secondarily by micro trauma. Thus, it is important to identify evidence of micro trauma, look for facial scarring that may be evidence of external trauma, and listen carefully for a history of trauma.

Range of Motion

Any of several types of devices can be used to measure the patient's total opening and lateral movements. It is important to note if the movements are pain free and if they can be done smoothly or with difficulty. The movement measurements are compared to averages such as 40 mm in opening and 10 mm in lateral directions. Do not simply measure but also analyze the potential cause and effect of any alteration in movement or form of movement. When a patient has limited movement to one side or demonstrates a deviation to one side upon opening, the clinician should determine which of the following causes pertain to this particular patient:

- Muscle spasm or tightness that interferes with normal movement
- Disc derangement, which can block normal movement
- Arthritic or adhesive stickiness of joint and joint tissue
- Fracture of condylar structures
- Tumor

- Degenerative disease
- Neurological etiology
- Avoidance of a particular tooth interference
- Normal movement because of developmental or birth defect of the joint apparatus
- A normal effect because of irregular condylar inclinations of right and left eminences

Joint Sounds

Either with a stethoscope or Doppler, the clinician can determine whether the crepitus sounds occur on excursive movement, on direct rotation, or both. This differentiation is helpful in evaluating whether the joint breakdown is an early or late type. There is evidence that most joint changes begin out on the lateral pole and may work themselves medially toward the medial pole. During excursive movements, the so-called joint loading takes place in areas other than the medial pole. Only during actual rotation does the loading take place in and around the medial pole. Through deductive reasoning, the clinician can conclude that, if crepitus is heard during rotation, the problem is more serious than if it is only heard on excursive movement.

Joint Palpation

Place gentle pressure on the area that demonstrates a slight depression as the patient opens, indicating the departure forward of the condyle and its lateral pole. Upon this pressure, the patient may feel tenderness if there has been damage to the lateral pole or there is inflammation of the retrodiscal tissues available for investigation by this same palpation.

Articulated Study Casts

The carefully and accurately made casts are mounted with a face bow and the very best beginning bite record available on the examination visit. A common error is to call this record a "centric relation record." It is often simply the bite du jour. The patient's muscle and joint condition may make it difficult, if not an insurmountable problem, to find the centric relation arc of closure until there has been therapy such as occlusal bite splint therapy. The longer the author has been in practice, the more the author has learned to rely on bite splint therapy to verify the centric relation arc of closure.

CR Analysis

One group of objectives is to evaluate the hinge movement, status of the joint and accompanying tissues, and the relative input of the muscles of mastication (degree of ease or difficulty) while finding the centric relation arc of closure. There is common acceptance that the centric relation arc of closure involves a seated and braced medial pole, a relaxed musculature, and a comfortable joint during hinge motion, even during joint loading. Please note the details of this procedure in chapter 4.

Digital Imaging

Digital photography, digital radiography, and various uses of CAT scan and CAD CAM technology are now not only commonplace but have become the standard of excellence in diagnostics and communication between patient, technician, and specialist. Throughout this text, uses and examples of these technologies will be illustrated. Clearly, patient education has been enhanced and restorative results have been made much more predictable by advanced digital technologies. Digital photography can enhance evaluation of the face, asymmetries, and dentition. Many diagnostic decisions are improved by analyzing the smile, lips at rest, profile, and extreme smile to determine the possible amount of lip movement. Chapter 8 details which views are critical and how to do the esthetic evaluation.

SAMPLE OCCLUSAL EXAMINATION FORM

The following occlusal examination form (figs. 1.1 a and b) is used by several visiting faculty of the Pankey Institute.

THE PATIENT'S UNDERSTANDING

After engaging the patient in co-discovery and collecting this kind of data, it is important to make sure the patient has an increased understanding of their own condition. This author likes to think that multiple potential "learning moments" can occur during the examination process. Throughout this book, there are examples of the clinician creating these "magical" learning moments. One frequently used technique is active listening during the comprehensive examination. By asking patients to clarify their understanding of each last completed step, the clinician stimulates extended dialogue. Oftentimes, the exam process takes an hour or more with conversation taking more of this time than data collection. The wise clinician makes time in the day's schedule for an extended appointment.

A definitive decision tree occurs as the clinician approaches the next step of diagnosis. Does the bulk of evidence for this particular patient weigh in more as an occlusal-muscle condition or as some related pathology or other condition of the temporomandibular joint apparatus? It is helpful for the patient to demonstrate where the pain occurs. Does the patient point with one finger to the joint? Or does the patient rub several

M. TEMPOROMANDIBULAR JOINT SYMPTOMS: DATE OF ONSET_____

R L	R L	R L	R L
☐ ☐ Negative	☐ ☐ Crepitus	☐ ☐ Hypomobility	☐ ☐ Upon Awakening
☐ ☐ Acute	☐ ☐ Clicking	☐ ☐ Chronic Subluxation	☐ ☐ When Eating
☐ ☐ Episodic	☐ ☐ Popping	☐ ☐ Spontaneous Dislocation	☐ ☐ When Yawning
☐ ☐ Chronic	☐ ☐ Painful	☐ ☐ Swallowing Discomfort	☐ ☐ When Sneezing
☐ ☐ Trauma	☐ ☐ Ear Ringing		☐ ☐ End of Day

N. MAXIMUM OPENING (AT MIDLINE) _____ **mm.**

☐ Normal	☐ Very Restricted	☐ Acute
☐ Limited	☐ Painful	☐ Chronic

O. MANDIBULAR DEFLECTION ON OPENING:

☐ None	☐ To Right - Then Left
☐ To Right	☐ To Left - Then Right
☐ To Left	

R   15 10 5 0 5 10 15 mm.

P. TEMPOROMANDIBULAR JOINT NOISE WITH MOVEMENT:

R L	R L	R L	R L
☐ ☐ Negative	☐ ☐ Crepitus	☐ ☐ Immediate	☐ ☐ Ausculative
☐ ☐ Vertical Opening	☐ ☐ Clicking	☐ ☐ Normal Range	☐ ☐ Audible
☐ ☐ Lateral Movement	☐ ☐ Popping	☐ ☐ Wide Range	☐ ☐ Very Loud

Q. TEMPOROMANDIBULAR JOINT RADIOGRAPHS:

IMAGE QUALITY :

R_____

L_____

R L	R L	R L	
☐ ☐ Concentric	☐ ☐ Reduced Joint Space	☐ ☐ Flattened Condyle	☐ ☐ Condyle Irregularities
☐ ☐ Condylar Protrusion	☐ ☐ Increased Joint Space	☐ ☐ Bony Lipping Condyle	
☐ ☐ Condylar Retrusion	☐ ☐ Fossae Irregularities	☐ ☐ Osteoporosis	
☐ ☐ Hypoplastic Condyle	☐ ☐ Bone Cyst	☐ ☐ Sclerosis Fossa	
☐ ☐ Hyperplastic Condyle	☐ ☐ Sclerosis Condyle	☐ ☐ Flattened Fossa	

R. TEMPOROMANDIBULAR JOINT PALPATION:

R L	R L	R L	R L
☐ ☐ Negative	☐ ☐ Sore	☐ ☐ Rubbing	☐ ☐ Without Movement
☐ ☐ Laterally	☐ ☐ Painful	☐ ☐ Irregular	☐ ☐ Opening
☐ ☐ From Auditory Canal	☐ ☐ Severe Pain	☐ ☐ Popping	☐ ☐ Closing

S. MUSCULAR PALPATION:

R L	R L	R L
☐ ☐ Negative	☐ ☐ Anterior Temporal (D)	☐ ☐ Sternomastoid (H)
☐ ☐ Lateral Pterygiud (A)	☐ ☐ Deep Masseter (E)	☐ ☐ Hyoid Area (I)
☐ ☐ Medial Pterygoid (B)	☐ ☐ Superficial Masseter (F)	☐ ☐ Occipital Area (J)
☐ ☐ Posterior Temporal (C)	☐ ☐ Digastric (G)	☐ ☐ Trapezius (K)

RED: Palpation
BLUE: Symptoms

RIGHT

LEFT

T. HEADACHES AND NECKACHES:

			R L
☐ Negative	☐ Vague Location	☐ No Medication	☐ ☐ Ocular
☐ Mild	☐ Variable Location	☐ Aspirin	☐ ☐ Aural
☐ Moderate	☐ Specific Location	☐ Tranquilizers	☐ ☐ Frontal
☐ Severe	☐ Minutes	☐ Anti-Depressants	☐ ☐ Sinus
☐ Migraine	☐ Hours	☐ Muscle Relaxants	☐ ☐ Parietal
☐ Chronic	☐ All Day	☐ Narcotics	☐ ☐ Temporal
☐ Episodic	☐ Days_____	☐ Ergotamines	☐ ☐ Occipital
			☐ ☐ Neck
			☐ ☐ Shoulder Area

HEADACHES PER MONTH_____

NECKACHES PER MONTH_____

U. OCCLUSAL HABITS

☐ Negative	☐ Anterior Bracing	☐ Morning Awareness	☐ Previous
☐ Suspected	☐ Clenching	☐ Resultant Sore Mouth	☐ Episodic
☐ Patient Aware	☐ Bruxism (Gnashing)	☐ Muscle Hypertrophy	☐ Current

V. EMOTIONAL STRESS LEVEL: CORNELL MEDICAL INDEX_____

☐ Negative	☐ Probable	☐ Sleep Loss	☐ Anxiety
☐ Questionable	☐ Pronounced	☐ Fatigue	☐ Frustration
☐ Suspected	☐ Severe	☐ Irritability	☐ Depression

W. POSSIBLE TREATMENT SEQUENCE:

☐ ___None	☐ ___Occlusal Splint	☐ ___Adrenocortical Injection
☐ ___Preventive Counseling	☐ ___Drug Therapy	☐ ___Orthodontic Consultation
☐ ___Limited Occlusal Adjustment	☐ ___Moist Heat	☐ ___Other TMJ Consultation
☐ ___Occlusal Equilibration	☐ ___Vapocoolant	☐ ___Medical Consultation
☐ ___Removable Prosthesis	☐ ___Muscle Exercises	☐ ___Neurological/Psychiatric
☐ ___Occlusal Reconstruction	☐ ___Local Anesthetic Injection	☐ ___Surgical Consultation

(a)

Figs. 1.1a and 1.1b. Occlusal examination form (Courtesy of Dr. Steve Hart and Dr. Carl Rieder).

PATIENT_____ AGE_____ DATE_____

A. MISSING TEETH:

R | 1 2 3 4 5 6 7 8 | 9 10 11 12 13 14 15 16 | L
32 31 30 29 28 27 26 25 | 24 23 22 21 20 19 18 17

B. FIRST CONTACT IN RETRUDED CONTACT POSITION (CENTRIC RELATION):

☐ Repeatable   ☐ Without Tenderness
☐ Questionable   ☐ Some Discomfort   R | 1 2 3 4 5 6 7 8 | 9 10 11 12 13 14 15 16 | L
☐ Undeterminable   ☐ Pain in R.C.P.   32 31 30 29 28 27 26 25 | 24 23 22 21 20 19 18 17

C. MANDIBULAR DISPLACEMENT (FROM RCP TO IP AT MIDLINE):

☐ None   ☐ Anterior ____mm.   ☐ To Right____ mm.
☐ Vertical_____mm.   ☐ To Left_____mm.

D. MANDIBULAR EXCURSIVE MOVEMENTS FROM INTERCUSPAL POSITION:

LATERAL GUIDANCE (WORKING)   BALANCING INTERFERENCES (NON-WORKING)

☐ None (Right Side)   ☐ Light (1)   ☐ Light (1)   ☐ None (Right Side)   ☐ Light (1)   ☐ Light (1)
☐ None (Left Side)   Right ☐ Moderate (2)   Left ☐ Moderate (2)   ☐ None (Left Side)   Right ☐ Moderate (2)   Left ☐ Moderate (2)
☐ Heavy (3)   ☐ Severe (3)   ☐ Severe (3)   ☐ Severe (3)

R | 1 2 3 4 5 6 7 8 | ← **RIGHT LATERAL MOVEMENT** → | 9 10 11 12 13 14 15 16 | L
32 31 30 29 28 27 26 25 | | 24 23 22 21 20 19 18 17

| 9 10 11 12 13 14 15 16 | L ← **LEFT LATERAL MOVEMENT** → R | 1 2 3 4 5 6 7 8 |
24 23 22 21 20 19 18 17 | | 32 31 30 29 28 27 26 25

E. ANTERIOR GUIDANCE:

☐ Key-in-Lock Facets
☐ Posterior Interference   R | 1 2 3 4 5 6 7 8 | 9 10 11 12 13 14 15 16 | L
☐ Adequate   32 31 30 29 28 27 26 25 | 24 23 22 21 20 19 18 17
☐ Proper anterior contact in C.O.
☐ Heavy anterior contact in C.O.
☐ No anterior contact in C.O.   RANGE OF MOTION
☐ Suspected Tongue Habits
☐ Verified Tongue Habits

☐ Deflection to Right   ☐ Deflection to Left

R └┴┴┴┴┴┴┴┘ L

F. ABNORMAL WEAR AND TOOTH FRACTURE:

☐ None   ☐ Opposing Porcelain (4)
☐ Light (1)   ☐ Fractured Filling (5)   R | 1 2 3 4 5 6 7 8 | 9 10 11 12 13 14 15 16 | L
☐ Moderate (2)   ☐ Fractured Cusp (6)   32 31 30 29 28 27 26 25 | 24 23 22 21 20 19 18 17
☐ Severe (3)   ☐ Split Tooth (7)

G. WIDENED PERIODONTAL SPACE:

☐ None
☐ Slight (1)   ☐ Uniform (4)   R | 1 2 3 4 5 6 7 8 | 9 10 11 12 13 14 15 16 | L
☐ Moderate (2)   ☐ Hour-Glass (5)   32 31 30 29 28 27 26 25 | 24 23 22 21 20 19 18 17
☐ Severe (3)   ☐ Occlusal Flaring (6)

H. ALVEOLAR BONE LOSS:

☐ None   ☐ Lamina Dura (5)
☐ Slight (1)   ☐ Horizontal (6)   R | 1 2 3 4 5 6 7 8 | 9 10 11 12 13 14 15 16 | L
☐ Moderate (2)   ☐ Vertical (7)   32 31 30 29 28 27 26 25 | 24 23 22 21 20 19 18 17
☐ Severe (3)   ☐ Infra Bony (8)
☐ Very Severe (4)   ☐ Furcation (9)

I. MISCELLANEOUS RESPONSE:

☐ None
☐ Hypercementosis (1)
☐ Osteosclerosis (2)
☐ Root Resorption (3)
☐ Pulpal Calcification (4)   R | 1 2 3 4 5 6 7 8 | 9 10 11 12 13 14 15 16 | L
☐ Exostosis (5)   32 31 30 29 28 27 26 25 | 24 23 22 21 20 19 18 17
☐ Cervical Erosion (6)
☐ Gingival Recession (7)
☐ Percussion Sensitivity (8)
☐ Thermal Sensitivity (9)

(b)   **OCCLUSAL-TMJ EXAMINATION**

Figs. 1.1a and 1.1b. *Continued*

fingers over a sore muscle area? The former likely indicates the condition originates in the joint, and the latter in the occlusal-muscle condition.

REFERENCES

Ash, M.M. (2006). Occlusion, TMDs, and dental education. *Head & Face Medicine*, Vol. 3.

Attanasio, R. (1991). Nocturnal bruxism and its clinical arrangement. *Dental Clinics of North America*, Vol. 35, pp. 245–252.

Baba, K. (1991). Influences of balancing-side interference on jaw function. *Kokubyo Gakkai Zasshi*, Vol. 58, pp. 118–137.

Belser, U.C., and Hannam, A.G. (1985). The influence of altered working-side occlusal guidance on masticatory muscles and related jaw movement. *Journal of Prosthetic Dentistry*, Vol. 53, pp. 406–413.

Braem, M., Lambrecht, P., and Vanherle, G. (1982). Stress induced cervical lesions. *Journal of Prosthetic Dentistry*, Vol. 67, pp. 718–722.

Campillo, M.J., Miralles, R., Santander, H., et al. (2008). Influencing of laterotrusive occlusal scheme on bilateral masseter EMG activity during clenching and grinding. *Cranio*, Vol. 26, pp. 263–273.

Clark, G.T., Tsukiyama, Y., Baba, K., et al. (1999). 67 years of experimental occlusal interferences studies: What have we learned? *Journal Prosthetic Dentistry*, Vol. 82, pp. 704–713.

Dejak, B., Mlotkowski, A., and Romanowicz, M. (2005). Finite element analysis of mechanism of cervical lesion formation in simulated molars during mastication and parafunction. *Journal of Prosthetic Dentistry*, Vol. 94, pp. 520–529.

Geering, A. (1974). Occlusal interferences and functional disturbance of the masticatory system. *Journal of Clinical Periodontology*, pp. 1–112.

Glaros, A.G., Forbes, M., Shanker, J., et al. (2000). Effect of parafunctional clenching on temporomandibular disorder pain and proprioceptive awareness. *Cranio*, Vol. 18, pp. 198–204.

Grippo, J.O. (1991). Abfractions: A new classification of hard tissue lesions of teeth. *Journal of Esthetic Dentistry*, Vol. 3, pp. 14–19.

Grippo, J.O., and Simring, M. (1995). Dental erosion revisited. *Journal of American Dental Association*, Vol. 126, pp. 619–620.

Kampe, T. (1987). Function and dysfunction of the masticatory system in individuals with intact and restored dentitions. A clinical, psychological and physiological study. *Swedish Dental Journal Supplement*, Vol. 42, pp. 1–68.

Kampe, T. Hannerz, H., and Strom, P. (1991). Five-year longitudinal recordings of functional variables of the masticatory system in adolescents with intact and restored dentitions. A comparative anamnestic and clinical study. *Acta Odontologica Scandinavia*, Vol. 49, pp. 239–246.

Kevilj, R., Mehulic, K., and Dundjer, A. (2007). Temporomandibular disorders and bruxism, Part 1. *Minerva Stomotologica*, Vol. 56, pp. 393–397.

Kuroe, T., et al. (2001). Biomechanical effects of cervical lesions and restoration on periodontally compromised teeth. *Quintessence International*, Vol. 32, pp. 111–118.

Lee, W.C., and Eakle, W.S. (1996). Stress induced cervical lesions: Review of advances in the past 10 years. *Journal of Prosthetic Dentistry*, Vol. 75, pp. 487–494.

Lytle, J.D. (1990). The clinician's index of occlusal disease: Definition, recognition, and management. *International Journal of Periodontics and Restorative Dentistry*, Vol. 10, pp. 103–123.

Lytle, J.D. (2001a). Occlusal disease revisited: Part I. Function and parafunction. *International Journal of Periodontics and Restorative Dentistry*, Vol. 21, pp. 264–271.

Lytle, J.D. (2001b). Occlusal disease revisited: Part II. *International Journal of Periodontics and Restorative Dentistry*, Vol. 21, pp. 272–279.

MacDonald, J.W., and Hannam, A.G. (1984). Relationship between occlusal contacts and jaw-closing muscle activity during tooth clenching: Part 1. *Journal of Prosthetic Dentistry*, Vol. 52, pp. 718–728.

Machado, N.A., Fonseca, R.B., Branco, C.A., et al. (2007). Dental wear caused by association between bruxism and gastroesophageal reflux disease: A rehabilitation report. *Journal of Applied Oral Science*, Vol. 15, pp. 327–333.

Madani, A.S., and Ahmadian-Yazdi, A. (2005). An investigation into the relationship between noncarious cervical lesions and premature contacts. *Journal of Craniomandibular Practice*, Vol. 23, pp. 10–15.

Moss, R.A., Villarosa, G.A., Cooley, J.E., et al. (1987). Masticatory muscle activity as a function of parafunctional, active and passive oral behavioral patterns. *Oral Rehabilitation*, Vol. 14, pp. 361–370.

Okamoto, A., Hayasaki, H., Nishijima, N., et al. (2000). Occlusal contacts during lateral excursions in children with primary dentition. *Dental Research*, Vol. 79, pp. 1890–1895.

Okeson, J.P. (1981). Etiology and treatment of occlusal pathosis and associated facial pain. *Journal of Prosthetic Dentistry*, Vol. 45, pp. 199–204.

Pegoraro, L., et al. (2005). Noncarious cervical lesions in adults. Prevalence and occlusal aspects. *Journal of the American Dental Association*, Vol. 136, pp. 1694–1700.

Pintado, M.R., et al. (2000). Correlation of noncarious cervical lesions size and occlusal wear in a single adult over a 14-year time span. *Journal of Prosthetic Dentistry*, Vol. 84, pp. 436–443.

Ratcliff, S., Becker, I., Quinn, L. (2001). Types and incidence of cracks in posterior teeth. *Journal of Prosthetic Dentistry*, Vol. 86, pp. 168–172.

Silvestri, A.R., Cohen, S.N., and Connolly, R.J. (1980). Muscle physiology during functional activities and parafunctional habits. *Journal of Prosthetic Dentistry*, Vol. 44, pp. 64–67.

Speck, J.E. (1988). The temporomandibular joint pain dysfunction syndrome. *Canadian Family Physician*, Vol. 34, pp. 1369–1374.

Spranger, H. (1995). Investigation into the genesis of angular lesions at the cervical region of teeth. *Quintessence International*, Vol. 26, pp. 149–154.

Wadhwa, S., and Kapila, S. (2008). TMJ disorders: Future innovations in diagnostics and therapeutics. *Journal of Dental Education*, Vol. 72, pp. 930–947.

Winter, R.R., and Allen, E.P. (2005). Restorative and periodontal considerations for the treatment of noncarious cervical lesions. *Advanced Esthetic and Interdisciplinary Dentistry*, Vol. 1, pp. 24–28.

Wood, W.W. (1987). A review of masticatory muscle function. *Journal of Prosthetic Dentistry*, Vol. 57, pp. 222–223.

Occlusal Parafunction and Temporomandibular Disorders: Neurobiological Considerations

Henry A. Gremillion, DDS, MAGD

The past several decades have heralded tremendous technologic and scientific advances in the field of dentistry. The demand for dental services has escalated dramatically as the general populace has gained an increased appreciation for the fact that quality oral health is a significant component of quality overall health. Scientific investigations have provided for an explosion of knowledge and enhanced understanding of numerous molecular biologic mechanisms underlying pathologic entities afflicting the dynamic stomatognathic system. Additionally, the unraveling of complexities of the peripheral and central neural substrates associated with health and pathology has prompted a broadened perspective in the evaluation, diagnosis, and treatment of patients with masticatory system dysfunction.

The form, function, and pathofunction of the dynamic masticatory system is one of the most fascinating, basic, and important areas of study in dentistry. Keen understanding of the many nuances associated with pathology is key to achieving sustainable comprehensive dental care for our patients. The goals of comprehensive dentistry include the following:

1. Maintain or return the patient to optimum oral health.
2. Promote anatomic and functional harmony between the various components of the masticatory system.
3. Encourage orthopedic stability.

Comprehensive Occlusal Concepts in Clinical Practice, by Irwin M. Becker
© 2011 Blackwell Publishing Ltd.

As the demand for dental care escalates, it must be kept in mind that pain and/or dysfunction is the most common reason for patients to seek care on a repeated basis. A broad scope survey of 45,711 households in the United States revealed that 22% of the U.S. population experienced orofacial pain on more than one occasion in a 6-month period (Lipton, Ship, and Larach-Robinson, 1993). While the most commonly experienced orofacial pain is odontogenic in nature, non-odontogenic orofacial pain such as temporomandibular disorder (TMD) is also common. Okeson (1996) defines TMD as "a collective term referring to a number of clinical problems involving the masticatory musculature, the temporomandibular joint(s), and associated structures or both." The prevalence of TMD-related pain has been reported to be 12% in the general population (Dworkin et al., 1990). Notably, more than 10 million Americans suffer from TMD-related complaints each year (NIH, 1996; Slavkin, 1996).

The etiology of TMD has been vigorously debated for many years. Heretofore, the diversity of opinion could be explained by the following:

1. A lack of precise definitions of the actual clinical conditions studied
2. Significant clinical/research bias
3. Lack of scientifically validated definitive cause and effect relationships

Additionally, various philosophies have viewed TMD in a narrow scope, promulgating single factors to be the primary cause of any or all of the subcategories of myogenous and arthrogenous pain and/or dysfunction.

The National Institute of Health Technology and Assessment Conference on Management of Temporomandibular Disorders fostered the more global biopsychosocial perspective (NIH, 1996). This concept views TMD to be a result of the dynamic interaction of biologic, psychologic, and social factors. However, a more purist stance would be to recognize the concept of bioburden, the effects of numerous factors affecting undue stress, and damage to a biological system. This perspective provides a template for delineation of signs and symptoms resulting from biopsychologic, biosocial, bioneuronal, biohormonal, and biomechanical burdens superceding the adaptive capacity of one or more of the components of the masticatory system, resulting in biomolecular changes.

What is universally agreed upon is that there exists a functional homeostatic balance between the various components of the masticatory system, including the teeth, periodontium (hard and soft tissue–supporting structures), masticatory and cervical musculature, temporomandibular joint structures, and the psyche of each individual. This balance within the masticatory system may be disrupted by a number of factors (bioburden) acting either alone or in combination resulting in the expression of signs and symptoms associated with TMD.

Basic science research has provided an enhanced understanding of pathogenesis, those cellular events and reactions and other pathologic mechanisms occurring in the development and maintenance or recurrence

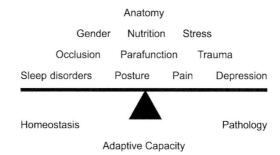

Anatomy

Gender   Nutrition   Stress

Occlusion   Parafunction   Trauma

Sleep disorders   Posture   Pain   Depression

Homeostasis   Pathology

Adaptive Capacity

Fig. 2.1. Endogenous and exogenous factors, which may disrupt the dynamic equilibrium (adaptive capacity) of the masticatory system, leading to the development and/or maintenance of temporomandibular disorder signs and symptoms. (Adapted from Parker, M.W. [1990]. A dynamic model of etiology in temporomandibular disorders. *Journal of the American Dental Association*, Vol. 120, pp. 283–290. Copyright © 1990 American Dental Association. All rights reserved. Adapted 2010 with permission of the American Dental Association.)

of TMD. Slavkin (1996) stated, "Understanding these interrelationships should improve how we promote health, reduce disease and enhance diagnosis and treatment." A model from Parker (1990) presents factors that may compromise the adaptability of the masticatory system and is represented in figure 2.1.

One of the areas of greatest contention relates to the association between occlusal factors as a causal role and TMD. Although occlusion has been recognized as an important etiologic or perpetuating cofactor, the degree to which it plays a role has not been definitively delineated. Few terms in dentistry are used in the broad context, as is *malocclusion*. Malocclusion is defined as "any deviation from acceptable contact of opposing dentitions or any deviation from normal occlusion" (MacDonald and Hannam, 1984). As a result, it is reasonable to ask, "What is normal occlusion?"

Analysis of 14 studies regarding the prevalence of malocclusion reveals that 42% of the population represent a Class I malocclusion, 23% exhibit Class II malocclusion, and 4% have a Class III malocclusion (Gremillion, 1995). Only 31% have what would be termed "normal occlusion." One may ask whether or not these occlusal relationships are truly aberrant or whether we are simply looking at static relationships in a dynamic orthopedic system.

The clinician is faced with the daunting task of determining on a case-specific basis whether occlusal factors are related to the patient's TMD symptoms. If a causal or cofactor role is determined, the clinician must then decide what the optimum occlusal contact relationship should be for the patient. The answers to these key questions are extremely important in the development of a case-specific, evidence-based treatment plan.

The conflicting information gleaned from the multitude of studies related to occlusion as a causal factor or utilization of occlusal therapy as a means of treating TMD may not reveal the total story. It is mandatory that the clinician/scientist consider the dynamic nature of the masticatory system. It has been stated that proper occlusion of the dentition occurs in a dynamic relationship with the oral and facial musculature, periodontium, supporting osseous framework, temporomandibular joints, and the enveloping neuromuscular system (MacDonald and Hannam, 1984). While it may be said that the manner in which teeth fit is important, what the individual does with his/her teeth may be more important when discussed in the context of relationship with TMD. The fact is that the masticatory system is an orthopedic system. It is well recognized that a common cause of pathology in orthopedic systems is overload, or mechanical stress.

The temporomandibular synovial system obeys the laws of orthopedics, as do other synovial systems. However, the masticatory system demonstrates a number of unique features that include the following:

- the right and left temporomandibular joints functioning as one unit held together by the dense cortical bone of the mandible,
- the articulating surfaces of each temporomandibular joint being fibrocartilaginous,
- the articular disc separating the temporomandibular joint into two compartments, allowing for complex movement,
- the temporomandibular joint being a ginglymoarthrodial (hinge-gliding) joint, and
- this unique articulation having a rigid endpoint, contact of the teeth, where the greatest forces are typically generated.

It is evident that the scientific literature has not convincingly demonstrated a definitive relationship between *static* occlusal factors and TMD. In contrast, *dynamic* occlusal function/parafunction has the potential to impact on multiple interfaces within the masticatory system, including the following:

- the tooth-to-tooth interface,
- the tooth/supporting structure interface,
- the TM joint interface, and
- muscle activity (functional and parafunctional).

Mechanical stresses at each of these interfaces have been shown to be associated with the potential to facilitate compromise in the integrity of tissues. Additionally, the clinician must consider the various case-specific factors that may affect each person's adaptability, such as the variable directions of muscular loading forces and the selective action of multiple dental and articular constraints influenced by the duration of load, the degree of load, and the individual's host resistance.

It is mandatory that we recognize the potential destructive effects of parafunction. In doing so, the triad of etiologic and/or perpetuating factors

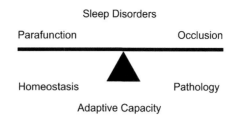

Fig. 2.2. Triad of occlusal parafunction.

related to occlusion, sleep disorders, and parafunction and their complex relationship must be considered (see figure 2.2).

Peripheral and central sensory and motor factors involved in masticatory system parafunction during waking and sleep times provide a complex integration of mechanisms with potential destructive effects.

Orofacial movement disorder (OMD) describes a spectrum of aberrations, both hyperactive and hypoactive, which involve the muscles of the orofacial complex innervated by the trigeminal, facial, and hypoglossal nerves (Clark and Ram, 2007). The most common types of OMD include sustained habitual forceful clenching (daytime and/or nighttime) and sleep bruxism (Clark and Ram, 2007).

Bruxism may be defined as the grinding or clenching of the teeth; however, stereotyped movements such as those associated with chewing are also considered under the broad domain of occlusal parafunction. These phenomena are produced by rhythmic contraction of the closure muscles of mastication, usually occurring without the individual's awareness. While the prevalence of some daytime parafunction is likely universal in society, the prevalence of sleep-related bruxism has been estimated at 5% to 90% of the total population. This disparity is likely related to the dependence on self-reporting and confounded by the fact that symptoms are not always associated with bruxism (Aggarwal et al., 2008; Glaros, 1981; Lavigne and Montplaisir, 1994; Ohayon, Li, and Guilleminault, 2001; Partinen, 1989).

In order to care for patients on a case-specific basis, it is incumbent on the dental professional to determine whether the patient presents with awake or sleep bruxism. Numerous daytime masticatory system parafunctional activities exist, including clenching; maladaptive posturing of the mandible; cheek, lip, and tongue biting; tooth tapping; and biting objects. Awake bruxism is typically a learned behavior. Therefore, management of awake bruxism is generally accomplished through awareness training (self-directed behavior modification) or through psychological retraining with biofeedback. Tooth grinding during waking hours is rare and, when present, typically associated with a neurological disorder or induced by medication (Lavigne et al., 2008).

Sleep bruxism has been defined in the ICDS-2 (AASM, 2005) as "an oral parafunction characterized by grinding or clenching of the teeth during sleep that is associated with an excessive (intense) sleep arousal activity." Sleep bruxism is classified as a parasomnia, a disorder of partial arousal during sleep that interferes with sleep stage transitions. A recognized sleep disorder, sleep bruxism appears to be primarily regulated centrally, not peripherally; however, peripheral factors may have some influence (Lobbezoo and Maeije, 2001). MacAluso et al. (1998) found that sleep bruxers experience a significantly higher number of transient arousals characterized by electroencephalographic (EEG) desynchronization. Therefore, based on current research, it is important for the dental professional to understand sleep stages and their relationship to sleep bruxism.

Humans spend 25% to 33% of their lives sleeping or at least trying to sleep. The benefits gained from a night's sleep vary greatly depending on a multitude of endogenous and exogenous factors. Sleep is a complex neurophysiologic process that is characterized by a regular and reversible behavioral state of perceptual disengagement from and unresponsiveness to the environment for varying periods of time. The immune system, mood, behavior, energy level, productivity, and cognitive ability are enhanced by appropriate quality and satisfactory quantity of sleep. Prolonged sleep deprivation, excessive sleep, or disrupted sleep patterns can profoundly compromise an individual's mental and cardiovascular status, as well as alter one's pain level defense (MacAluso et al., 1998). Sleep disruption and sleep disorders have a profound effect on individuals and on society. An awareness of specific sleep disorders, as well as their diagnosis and management, is more important than ever in the practice of medicine and dentistry (Moldofsky, 1993).

The orafacial region is one of the most common places in which pain is experienced. It is not uncommon for patients with chronic or recurrent pain to report poor sleep quality with a reduction in the perceived quantity of sleep. Importantly, it has been suggested that nonrestorative sleep is frequently a secondary complaint of pain patients (Shapiro and Dement, 1993). Riley et al. (2001) reported that 50% to 70% of patients with chronic pain experience sleep disturbances. Of 128 chronic orofacial pain patients randomly evaluated, 77% reported a reduced sleep quantity since pain onset (Morin and Wade, 1998).

To understand the impact of compromised sleep, one must first understand sleep architecture and the differences between the various stages of sleep. Utilization of electroencephalograms allows for enhanced understanding of normal and abnormal sleep stage variations in brain activity. The sleep architecture of non–rapid eye movement (N-REM) and rapid eye movement (REM) sleep stages is depicted in figure 2.3.

Recent studies have elucidated the genesis of sleep bruxism to be associated with motor systems and autonomic-cardiac interactions. Sleep laboratory studies have demonstrated that bruxism occurs during light sleep (Stages 1 and 2). Most episodes of sleep bruxism are apparently related to brief cardiac and brain reactivations (micro-arousals) lasting from 3 to 15 seconds (Lavigne et al., 2007). Major risk factors for sleep bruxism that may

---

Sleep Architecture

A. **Non-Rapid Eye Movement (N-REM) Sleep provides rest for the mind.**
   i. Stage 1 is a transitional stage that accounts for approximately 5% of one's sleep.
   ii. Stage 2 makes up approximately 50% of one's sleep.
   iii. Stage 3 ⎤
                In combination with Stage 4, Stage 3 makes up approximately 25% of one's sleep and is referred to as slow wave sleep, delta sleep or restorative sleep.
   iv. Stage 4 ⎦
      - *Growth hormone is released mainly at night in association with slow wave sleep.*
      - *T-cell and lymphocyte function is enhanced by slow wave sleep.*
      - *Serotonin levels are highest during slow wave sleep.*

B. **Rapid Eye Movement (REM) sleep (20% of one's sleep) provides rest for the body and is known as the dream state.**

   There is a lack of autonomic nervous system control during REM sleep which may represent a risk period for health and may be a precipitating factor in nocturnal death.

Fig. 2.3. Sleep architecture of normal stages of sleep.

cause sleep fragmentation, sleep-stage shifts, and micro-arousals include nicotine, caffeine, and/or alcohol use; anxiety; systemic factors such as peptic ulcer disease and gastroesophogeal reflux; and sleep disorders. Sleep apnea has been associated with bruxism with an odds ratio of 8, while snoring demonstrated an odds ratio of 4 (Lavigne et al., 2007).

Sleep-related gastroesophageal reflux disease is quite common in the general adult population. The impact on the individual's general dental health relative to erosion, decay, and compromised periodontal health can be significant. Sleep-related gastroesophageal reflux disease is associated with the regurgitation of stomach contents, which are extremely caustic (pH <4). Normal oral pH is approximately 6.75. When this erosive process is concurrent with an abrasive process, such as sleep-related bruxism, loss of tooth structure can progress at a rapid rate. The erosion associated with gastroesophogeal reflux disease, overlaid on abrasion from occlusal parafunction (awake and sleep-related bruxism), can be seen in figures 2.4 and 2.5.

The absolute pathophysiology of sleep bruxism is yet to be determined. It is theorized to be a neuromotor dysregulation disorder in which there

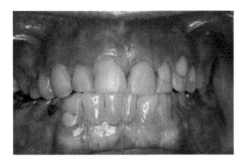

Fig. 2.4. Frontal view of erosion and abrasion.

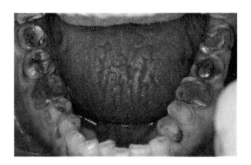

Fig. 2.5. Intra-oral view of erosion and abrasion.

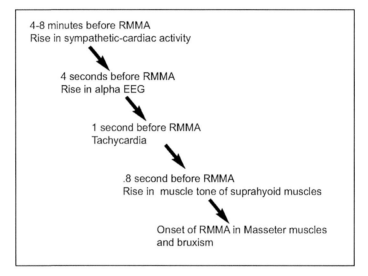

Fig. 2.6. Bruxism: autonomic-cardiac relationship with rhythmic masticatory muscle activity (RMMA).

is an EEG activation and motor neuron excitability resulting from neuro-chemical processes. However, the role of peripheral sensory inputs (periodontal) and cognitive-behavioral factors (stress, anxiety, and personality) must also be considered.

Further evidence of the relationship between sleep bruxism and micro-arousals was identified by Kato et al. (2003). They found that experimentally induced rhythmic masticatory muscle activity (RMMA) related to micro-arousals were followed by bruxism in over 70% of trials in sleep bruxism subjects and not in controls. The association between an elevation in sympathetic tone or autonomic-cardiac interactions and RMMA was clearly determined in an eloquent study by Lavigne et al. (2007), as demonstrated in figure 2.6. Limb movements (body disturbances of sleep) are associated with RMMA and the microarousals.

What is the impact of bruxism on the masticatory system? Review of the literature regarding oral parafunction and TMD provides insight as to a potential relationship between what goes on at the tops of the teeth and TMD. Carlsson, Egermark, and Magnusson (2003) reported data collected in a 20-year longitudinal study. At baseline, 402 randomly selected 7-, 11-, and 15-year-old subjects were evaluated for occlusal factors, oral parafunction, tooth wear, and TMD. Twenty years later, 320 subjects were assessed for the same variables. Logistic regression indicated that childhood parafunction (bruxism, tooth clenching, nocturnal grinding, and nail biting) were predictors of the same oral parafunction 20 years later. They also reported that childhood parafunction and an Angle Class II malocclusion were predictors of tooth wear in adulthood. Magnusson, Egermark, and Carlsson (2005) reported that evaluation of this same study population at the 4–5-, 10-, and 20-year marks revealed significant correlation between bruxism and TMD symptoms.

Another recent publication (Gesch et al., 2005) reported on the association between morphologic occlusion and functional occlusal factors and TMD symptoms. In this study, 4,310 subjects were evaluated. No specific occlusal factor was found to be significantly associated with TMD symptoms. However, parafunction demonstrated a positive relationship to TMD symptoms (odds ratio 3.4).

It is clear that degenerative temporomandibular joint disease is the result of maladaptation to increased joint loading (de Bont and Stegenga, 1993; Milam, 1995; Milam, Zardeneta, and Schmitz, 1998; Westesson and Rohlin, 1984). An oxidative-stress mechanism involving free radicals and other chondrodestructive factors has been recently been suggested (Milam, Zardeneta, and Schmitz, 1998; Saxton, Donnelly, and Roper, 1994). The changes that take place at the neuromuscular interface must also be appreciated. Isometric contraction such as that associated with clenching the teeth has specific local effects, including increased pressure within the muscle, obstruction of blood flow, decreased oxygen saturation, decreased glycogen saturation, and impaired removal of catabolic by-products. Free radicals have been implicated in exercise-induced muscle damage (Saxton, Donnelly, and Roper, 1994). Muscle overuse and eccentric contractions have been demonstrated to cause muscle fiber damage with associated edema/effusion. A local release of mediator substance P and calcitonin gene–related peptide into the extracellular space might signal other cells (mast cells) to initiate humoral or cellular-based inflammation and set the stage for peripheral sensitization of nociceptors. The pain associated with this form of postexercise muscle soreness generally peaks at 3–4 days postparafunctional episode.

It is evident that the scientific literature has not convincingly demonstrated a definitive relationship between static occlusal factors and TMD. TMD represents a multifaceted/multifactorial group of conditions that share common signs and symptoms. Although a multitude of factors have been theorized to initiate TMD, there exist individual variables that may potentially play a causal role alone or in combination with other factors. There are many theorized etiologic factors yet to be scientifically validated. The true determining factor(s) may be related to the individual's host resistance or adaptive capacity.

If we are to take an evidence-based view of occlusion and TMD, we must be able to differentiate between an occlusal contact and an occlusal interference. It is mandatory that we recognize the potential destructive effects of parafunction. Therefore, it may be more appropriate to view TMD cases in which occlusal function serves as a significant factor in TMD as a *maladaptive* occlusion. This term takes into consideration peripheral and central sensory and motor factors involved in masticatory system pathofunction on a case-specific basis and is supported by the recognized effects of mechanical stress on the stomatognathic system.

REFERENCES

Aggarwal, V.R., McBeth, J., Zakrzewska, J.M., et al. (2008). Are reports of mechanical dysfunction in chronic orofacial pain related to somatization? A population based study. *European Journal of Pain*, Vol. 12, pp. 501–507.

American Academy of Sleep Medicine (2005). *International Classification of Sleep Disorders*, 2nd ed. Westchester, IL: Author.

Carlsson, G.E., Egermark, I., Magnusson, T. (2003). Predictors of bruxism, other oral parafunctions, and tooth wear over a 20-year follow-up period. *Journal of Orofacial Pain*, Vol. 17, pp. 50–57.

Clark, G.T., and Ram, S. (2007). Four oral motor disorders: Bruxism, dystonia, dyskinesia and drug-induced dystonic extrapyramidal reactions. *Dental Clinics of North American*, Vol. 51, pp. 225–243.

de Bont, L.G., and Stegenga, B. (1993). Pathology of temporomandibular joint internal derangement and osteoarthrosis. *International Journal of Oral Maxillofacial Surgery*, Vol. 22, pp. 71–74.

Dworkin, S.F., Huggins, K.H., LeResche, L., et al. (1990). Epidemiology of signs and symptoms of temporomandibular disorders: Clinical signs in cases and controls. *Journal of the American Dental Association*, Vol. 120, pp. 273–281.

Gesch, D., Bernhardt, O., Mack, F., et al. (2005). Association of malocclusion and functional occlusion with subjective symptoms of TMD in adults: Results of the Study of Health in Pomerania (SHIP). *Angle Orthodontics*, Vol. 75, pp. 183–190.

Glaros, A.G. (1981). Incidence of diurnal and nocturnal bruxism. *Journal of Prosthetic Dentistry*, Vol. 45, pp. 545–549.

Gremillion, H.A. (1995). TMD and maladaptive occlusion: Does a link exist? *Journal of Craniomandibular Practice*, Vol. 13, pp. 205–206.

Kato, T., Montplaisir, J.Y., Guitard, F., et al. (2003). Evidence that experimentally induced sleep bruxism is a consequence of transient arousal. *Journal of Dental Research*, Vol. 82, pp. 284–288.

Lavigne, G.J., Huynh, N., Kato, T., et al. (2007). Genesis of sleep bruxism: Motor and autonomic-cardiac interactions. *Archives of Oral Biology*, Vol. 52, pp. 381–384.

Lavigne, G.J., Khoury, S., Abe S., et al. (2008). Bruxism physiology and pathology: An overview for clinicians. *Journal of Oral Rehabilitation*, Vol. 35, pp. 476–494.

Lavigne, G.J., and Montplaisir, J.Y. (1994). Restless legs syndrome and sleep bruxism: Prevalence and associations among Canadians. *Sleep*, Vol. 17, pp. 739–743.

Lipton, J.A., Ship, J.A., and Larach-Robinson, D. (1993). Estimated prevalence and distribution of reported orofacial pain in the United States. *Journal of the American Dental Association*, Vol. 124, pp. 115–121.

Lobbezoo, F., and Maeije, M. (2001). Bruxism is mainly regulated centrally, not peripherally. *Journal of Oral Rehabilitation*, Vol. 28, pp. 1085–1091.

MacAluso, G.M., Guerra, P., Di Giovanni, G., et al. (1998). Sleep bruxism is a disorder related to periodic arousals during sleep. *Journal of Dental Research*, Vol. 77, pp. 565–573.

MacDonald, J.W., and Hannam, A.G. (1984). Relationship between occlusal contacts and jaw-closing muscle activity during tooth clenching: Part I. *Journal of Prosthetic Dentistry*, Vol. 52, pp. 718–728.

Magnusson, T., Egermark, I., and Carlsson, G.E. (2005). A prospective investigation over two decades on signs and symptoms of temporomandibular disorders and associated variables: A final summary. *Acta Odontal Scandinavia*, Vol. 63, pp. 99–109.

Milam, S.B. (1995). Articular disk displacements and degenerative temporomandibular joint disease. In: *Temporomandibular Disorders and Related Pain Conditions* (eds. B.J. Sessle, P.S. Bryant, and R.A. Dionne), pp. 89–112. Seattle: IASP Press.

Milam, S.B., Zardeneta, G., and Schmitz, J.P. (1998). Oxidative stress and degenerative temporomandibular joint disease: A proposed hypothesis. *Journal of Oral Maxillofacial Surgery*, Vol. 56, pp. 214–223.

Moldofsky, H. (1993). Sleep and musculoskeletal pain. In: *Progress in Fibromyalgia and Myofascial Pain* (eds. H. Voeroy and H. Merskey), pp. 137–148. Amsterdam: Elsevier.

Morin, C.M., and Wade, J. (1998). Self-reported sleep and mood disturbance in chronic pain patients. *Clinical Journal of Pain*, Vol. 14, pp. 311–314.

National Institute of Health Technology and Assessment Conference. (1996). Management of temporomandibular disorders. *NIH Technology Assessment Statement*, Apr 29–May 1, pp. 1–31.

Ohayon, M.M., Li, K.K., and Guilleminault, C. (2001). Risk factors for sleep bruxism in the general population. *Chest*, Vol. 119, pp. 53–61.

Okeson, J.P. (1996). Differential diagnosis and management considerations of temporomandibular disorders. In: *Orofacial Pain: Guidelines for Assessment, Diagnosis and Management*, pp. 113–184. Chicago: Quintessence.

Parker, M.W. (1990). A dynamic model of etiology in temporomandibular disorders. *Journal of the American Dental Association*, Vol. 120, pp. 283–290.

Partinen M. (1989). Epidemiology of sleep disorders. In: *Principles and Practice of Sleep Medicine*, 2nd ed. (eds. M.H. Kryger, T. Roth, and W.C. Dement), pp. 437–452. Philadelphia: W.B. Saunders.

Riley, J.L., Benson, M.B., Gremillion, H.A., et al. (2001). Sleep disturbance in orofacial pain patients: Pain related or emotional distress? *Journal of Craniomandibular Practice*, Vol. 19, pp. 106–113.

Saxton, J.M., Donnelly, A.E., and Roper, H.P. (1994). Indices of free-radical-mediated damage following maximum voluntary eccentric and concentric muscular work. *European Journal of Applied Physiology and Occupational Physiology*, Vol. 8, pp. 189–193.

Shapiro, C.M., and Dement, W.C. (1993). ABC of sleep disorders: Impact and epidemiology of sleep disorders. *British Medical Journal*, Vol. 306, pp. 1604–1607.

Slavkin, H.C. (1996). Lifetime of motion: Temporomandibular joints. *Journal of the American Dental Association*, Vol. 127, pp. 1093–1098.

Westesson, P.L. and Rohlin, M. (1984). Internal derangement related to osteoarthrosis in temporomandibular joint autopsy specimens. *Oral Surgery, Oral Medicine, Oral Pathology, Oral Radiology and Endodontology*, Vol. 57, pp. 17–22.

3

The Masticatory System: Orthopedic Considerations in Function and Pathofunction

Henry A. Gremillion, DDS, MAGD
Christopher J. Spencer, DDS

The human masticatory system is a dynamic orthopedic system that is dramatic in its complexity. Dr. Peter E. Dawson has stated that dentists are the physicians of the masticatory system. We concur wholeheartedly. Due to the integration of innervations in the head and neck and the interdependence between cranial and cervical components in routine function, it may be stated that dentists must be physicians of the masticatory system and beyond.

To establish optimum masticatory system health, temporomandibular joint (TM joint) stability, muscle comfort and optimal function, and occlusal stability, anatomic and functional harmony must be appreciated. In practical terms, masticatory system health is equated to a great extent with orthopedic stability. The purpose of this chapter is to explore how orthopedic stability within the masticatory system is maintained or lost through dynamic interactions between various components.

Several key features make the masticatory system unique compared to other synovial joint systems. The right and left side TM joints function as one unit because the mandible is fused at the midline. If one TM joint moves, the other is affected and cannot function in an independent fashion. Since the TM joint is a ginglymoarthrodial (hinge and gliding) joint, it can function in an almost infinite number of positions within its normal range of motion. Significantly, as highlighted in chapter 2, the masticatory system displays a rigid end point at one end range of movement. When the mandible is closed, it is irrevocably stopped by contact of the teeth, except in

Comprehensive Occlusal Concepts in Clinical Practice, by Irwin M. Becker
© 2011 Blackwell Publishing Ltd.

the completely edentulous individual. This feature, unique to synovial joint systems, is key to understanding the form, function, and pathofunction of the TM joint since the majority of forces are typically applied to the system through the tops of the teeth.

Since the masticatory system is dynamic, not static, and exemplifies a complex integration between various components, all components must be evaluated during the comprehensive examination. Key components include the teeth, hard and soft tissue–supporting structures, masticatory and cervical musculature, and the TM joints.

Unfortunately, many studies related to causal factors and the development of pathology in this dynamic orthopedic system have looked at static or passive relationships. In truth, when the clinician is evaluating the masticatory system for compromised function such as associated with a multitude of muscle-based and joint-based disorders, how teeth fit may be important, but what people do with their teeth may be more important.

Intuitively, it is known that the primary reason orthopedic systems break down is due to orthopedic overload—excessive force that exceeds the adaptive capacity of the system. In the masticatory system, this most likely occurs during parafunctional activity (activities beyond normal function), as highlighted in chapter 2.

It is clear that long-term excessive load has detrimental consequences. Forces generated within the system during function and parafunction are distributed throughout the system through the teeth. The following interfaces are affected by the distribution of forces:

- The tooth-to-tooth interface
- The dentin-to-pulp interface
- The tooth-to–supporting structure interface
- The tooth-to-neuromuscular interface
- The tooth-to–TM joint interface

The effects of direction, duration, degree of load, and host resistance must be considered on a case-specific basis.

Pathenogenesis is defined as "the cellular events and reactions and other pathologic mechanisms occurring in the development of disease" (Milam, 2005). Many factors must be considered as we assess and analyze form, function, and pathofunction. Principally, we must appreciate the changes that may occur at the different interfaces of occlusion as a result of forces generated. These forces have the potential to tip the balance from adaptability to pathology.

THE TOOTH-TO-TOOTH INTERFACE

Wear of the dentition may be the result of a number of factors, including abnormal occlusal contacts, oral pH, disorders of the dentition such enamel dysplasia or hyperplasia, loss of posterior support, and changes related to aging, environmental factors, dietary factors, and cultural habits. Excessive forces applied at the tooth-to-tooth interface may be demonstrated as wear or fracture.

Changes at the cementoenamel junction have also been suggested to result from excessive forces applied to the dentition. Abfractive lesions, defined as stress-induced lesions resulting from hyperfunction and parafunction that can be further exacerbated by other factors such as erosion-corrosion and/or toothbrush or dentifrice abrasion, have been reported in the scientific literature (Grippo, 1991; Owens and Gallien, 1995). It has been suggested that abnormal occlusal mechanical stress may initiate disruption of the hydroxyapatite crystals in the cervical region of the tooth. Other authors describe the relationship between flexure of cusps and cervical lesions during excessive occlusal load, suggesting that these forces generate large areas of concentrated stress in the cervical regions of teeth. Persistent loading of cusps leads to flexure, which can lead to the breakdown of the bonds between hydroxyapatite crystals with the consequent loss of tooth structure (Rees, 2002). Abfractive lesions have been shown to be complex multifactorial phenomena; however, excessive occlusal load certainly must be considered as a contributing factor.

Excessive occlusal forces have long been implicated in vertical root fracture. Demographic studies have shown that the most common teeth implicated in vertical fracture are mandibular first and second molars (42% of all fractures) and maxillary premolars (23.35%). Cohen et al. (2006) concluded from a study of 227 teeth with vertical root fractures that excessive force, in combination with weakened coronal structure, was the most common cause of vertical fracture.

Gao, Yin, and Wu (2001) concluded from another study that excessive occlusal forces of a repetitive nature in specific chewing patterns would likely produce vertical root fractures. Yeh (1997), in a series of 46 cases of root fracture occurring in 51 non-endodontically treated teeth reported that these fractures occurred in individuals 40 years and older 96% of the time. The author concluded that a stress fatigue process was the etiology of these vertical fractures.

DENTIN-TO-PULP INTERFACE

The effects of traumatic occlusion can also be expressed in the dental pulp. Pressure applied to the occlusal surface of the tooth has been shown to result in an increased fluid flow in the dentinal tubules and a corresponding increase of activity in pulpal sensory nerves (Markowitz, 1993; Brännström, 1966). Pulpal axons display increased activity of substances P and CGRP, neuromodulators, which are key biochemical markers of pain (Vandevska-Radunovic et al., 1992; Kviinnsland et al., 1992).

Mechanical stress, associated with occlusal forces, has also been shown to affect the vascular supply to the dental pulp (Jafarzadeh, 2009). Regular use of chewing gum has been shown to create vasoconstriction of the apical vascular supply to the pulp with a compensation of increased capillary blood flow in the pulp tissue itself (Loginova and Ivanova, 2008). Thus, it can be safely stated that excessive occlusal load leads to vascular, cellular, and neurologic changes in the dental pulp tissue.

It appears that odontoblasts recognize and respond to physiologic occlusal stimulation. Occlusal forces affect the activity of odontoblasts, resulting in secretion of proteins such as precollagen in the dentinal tubules. The odontoblastic processes extend further into dentinal tubules in the occlusal regions of the tooth (near the cusps) than in the cervical region (Sato et al., 2009).

THE TOOTH-TO–SUPPORTING STRUCTURE INTERFACE

It must be recognized that occlusal forces are important for the maintenance of the human periodontium. When occlusal forces are absent, the alveolar bone and supporting structures atrophy. The supporting structures of the teeth are in a dynamic equilibrium. Occlusal load applied through the long axis helps to maintain the periodontal ligament, alveolar bone, vascular supply, and collagen fiber support.

However, excessive load may result in degradation in the same tissues. As early as 1961, Muhlemann and Herzog found occlusal trauma was implicated in degenerative changes in the periodontal ligament. A localized vasculitis was observed that was also associated with a disorganization of periodontal ligament cells and collagen fibers. These microscopic changes in the periodontal ligament lead to increased tooth mobility. If the trauma was sufficiently severe, necrosis of collagen fibers occurred and even hyalinization of the periodontal ligament.

The fine line between acceptable occlusal loads and trauma-inducing loads may be related to the matricellular protein periostin. This protein was originally discovered in the periodontal ligament but has now been widely identified in skin, muscle, and cardiac tissues (involved in cardiac muscle healing and valvular remodeling). Periostin plays a fundamental part in tissue remodeling and interacts with other proteins that are associated with cell adhesion, cell proliferation, and cell differentiation (Kudo et al., 2007). Occlusal load applied to teeth helps to maintain periostin levels. When periostin is absent in genetic animal studies, periodontal defects occurred under normal occlusal loads. If the occlusal loads were removed, the periodontal defects were "rescued" (Rios et al., 2008). Periostin has been implicated in collagen fibrinogenesis (Hamilton, 2008). This makes periostin a very interesting biomarker since periodontal breakdown involves the disorganization of periodontal cells, inability to repair, lack of fibroblast differentiation to heal affected areas, and collagen breakdown.

Fibroblasts have been found to play a role in alveolar bone breakdown due to their ability to produce cytokines, well-known inflammatory mediators. Cytokine IL-1 has been identified in gingival crevicular fluid in patients with periodontal disease and has been shown to elicit bone resorption. Periodontal ligament cells also release IL-6, which has been demonstrated to be involved in bone metabolism in periodontal disease and orthodontic tooth movement. IL-8 also can result in periodontal destruction and alveolar bone resorption through osteoclastogenesis (Shimizu et al., 1992). Occlusal trauma can induce specific changes in the distribution and shape of nerve terminals in the periodontal ligament, which are adjacent to the fibroblasts producing mediators. When these chemical mediators interact with the immune system, periodontal destruction may ensue (Sodeyama, 1996).

The relationship between occlusion and the supporting structures of the teeth is complex and multifaceted. Occlusal overload can affect this system, shifting the balance from an adaptive state to a pathologic state.

THE TOOTH-TO-NEUROMUSCULAR INTERFACE

The dentition is a highly sensitive touch and pressure organ of the somatic sensory system of the orofacial region. This sensory system is expressed through the teeth to the periodontal ligament. The innervations for the touch receptors in the periodontal ligament and the muscle spindles (stretch and length receptors) of the masticatory muscles are provided by the mesencephalic nucleus (Jerge, 1963). Occlusal contacts affect all of the muscles of mastication, but the contraction masseter and temporalis muscles are mostly dependent on contact of posterior teeth. Anterior teeth contacts have demonstrated inhibitory influences on these same muscles (Sheikholeslam and Riise, 1983). The control of the muscles in masticatory activities is refined and precisely controlled. The recruitment patterns of the muscles (specific motor units of each muscle) determine the direction of the load within the periodontal and TM joint regions. The number, position, and bilateral of occlusal contacts has a major impact on the amount and direction of forces applied by the muscles of mastication.

There are a number of occlusal factors that should be considered in respect to their influence on the muscles of mastication. These factors have the potential to influence pain and dysfunction.

- Lateral deviation in slide from muscle relaxed (centric relation or adapted centric relation) position to maximum intercuspation
- Lateral guidance on posterior teeth
- Distalizing forces
- Balancing interferences
- Protrusive guidance on posterior teeth

Lateral Deviation in Slide

The amount and direction of slide from muscle relaxed (centric relation or adapted centric relation) position to maximum intercuspation is examined by comparing the mandibular midline to the maxillary midline relationship in centric relation occlusion, and the initial centric relationship contact to the relationship in maximum intercuspal position. The slide can occur in three dimensions: vertical, anterior-posterior, and lateral. Significant lateral slides can create larger potential shearing forces to the attachment of the articular disc at the lateral pole of the condyle than vertical or anterior posterior slides. If the attachment of the articular disc to the condyle is compromised, the lateral pterygoid muscle, which inserts into the condylar fovea and the anteriomedial aspect of the articular disc (superior belly of the lateral pterygoid), can move the articular disc in an approximately 45-degree anteriomedial direction. The inferior belly of the lateral pterygoid muscle contracts during opening, protrusive, and contralateral movements of the mandible. The superior belly is active during closure of the mandible only with an eccentric (lengthening while contracting) type of contraction (Mahan et al., 1983).

Lateral Guidance on Posterior Teeth

Different types of occlusal contacts elicit different responses from the muscles of mastication. Anterior contact during vertical closure produces less muscle activity than posterior contact. Anterior contact in lateral excursions has an inhibitory effect on muscle contraction (Williamson and Lundquist, 1983).

An eloquent study by Korioth and Hannam (1994) demonstrated that the number, position of posterior contacts, and presence of balancing occlusal contacts affected muscle recruitment patterns. The recruitment of different muscles and different motor units within muscles determine the direction of load applied through the teeth to the periodontal ligament. Reaction forces during parafunctional activity in maximum intercuspation were the highest on most posterior teeth and decreased in teeth in more anterior regions. It was found to be the least in the premolar region and intermediate in the canine region. Reaction forces with group function with a balancing contact were found to be highest in the most posterior locations on the working side. The forces were least at the ipsilateral canine. The balancing side molar contact was equal in intensity to the highest force on the working molar. Reactive forces involving only balancing side contacts provided the highest of all clenching forces in muscle recruitment patterns (Korioth and Hannam, 1994). It is clear that different types of occlusal contacts provide large variations in masticatory muscle recruitment patterns.

Distalizing Forces

The condyle while seated in the glenoid fossa normally rests on the articular disc with forces directed in a superior, anterior, medial direction. If the condyle is forced distally, it can compress the highly vascularized and innervated retrodiscal tissues in the posterior aspect of the TM joint with resultant pain and inflammation. Distalizing forces may be the result of infringement on the envelope of function via tooth movement or bulky restorations. These same types of forces can be generated in a natural dentition in an Angle Class II canine relationship. During lateral movement to the working side, the mandibular canine can rest against the distal incline (ridge blade) of the maxillary canine, forcing the mandible in a posterior (distalizing) direction. If distalizing contacts are evident during a patient examination, the posterior temporalis and/or the posterior digastrics muscle may be painful due to a conscious or subconscious resulting attempt to avoid the uncomfortable contact since these muscles function to retrude the mandible.

Balancing Interferences

Posterior balancing side guidance can occur in either the functional range or in crossover (mandibular canines beyond the maxillary canines). These types of interferences can provoke muscular hyperactivity in the superficial masseter, deep masseter, the anterior temporalis, and the medial pterygoid muscles. Excessive occlusal forces can cause breakdown of many different aspects of the masticatory system, including fractured teeth, mobile teeth, tooth migration, fracture restorations, sore muscles of mastication, and degenerative changes in the TM joint.

Protrusive Guidance on Posterior Teeth

Protrusive guidance on posterior teeth rather than on anterior teeth is associated with a loss of the inhibitory effect on masticatory muscle activity provided by anterior tooth contact. This situation may result in masticatory muscle fatigue and pain affecting the superficial masseter, deep masseter, anterior temporalis, and/or the medial pterygoid.

Dysfunctional occlusal contacts may contribute to masticatory muscle hyperactivity. There are three types of muscle contraction: concentric, isometric, and eccentric. During prolonged isometric contraction of muscles (activation of both flexor and extensor muscles), a number of local effects are exhibited. The contractile forces generate increased pressure within the muscle, with the resultant obstruction of blood flow, decreased oxygen saturation, decreased glycogen saturation, and impaired removal of catabolic by-products.

Eccentric type of muscle contraction demonstrates muscle fiber damage with even moderate hyperactivity. Edema and effusion can last for up to 80 days, while pain only lasts for 3 to 5 days. As muscles relax and blood flows freely back into the body of the muscle, oxygen reperfusion takes place with the likelihood of reactive oxygen species occurring (free radical formation), which can damage the muscle tissue (Saxton, Donnelly, and Roper, 1994).

Myositis, an acute inflammatory muscle condition, occurs following localized muscle injury or infection. Onset is often the result of prolonged or unaccustomed use, including masticatory parafunction. This condition is associated with pain during mandibular movement and concomitant limitation in the range of motion. Myositis may affect a single muscle or may affect multiple muscles of mastication with a generalized presentation. The inflammation is expressed as edema (puffy muscle presentation) and pain.

THE TOOTH-TO-TM JOINT INTERFACE

The TM joint is irrevocably connected to the rest of the masticatory system and the teeth. All forces that are applied to the masticatory system are also applied to the TM joint as well.

Orthopedic systems typically break down from overload (biomechanical stress). The two main risk factors for osteoarthritis are increasing age (risk increases with each decade) and joint loading that exceeds the adaptive capacity of the joint. Both of these risk factors affect the chondrocytes' ability to maintain the articular surface (Marting et al., 2004). The masticatory system and the TM joint are no exception. In the healthy TM joint, the articular disc is interposed between the condyle and the glenoid fossa. The TM joint, masticatory muscles, and teeth with their supporting structures work together in an intricate neuronally orchestrated manner. If excessive prolonged force is applied, degenerative changes can occur.

Degenerative joint disease is the result of maladaptation due to increased joint loading (Westesson and Rohlin, 1984; deBont and Stegenga, 1993). Degenerative joint disease is a chronic inflammatory or noninflammatory disease resulting in joint deformity caused by degenerative changes in the articular cartilage, fibrous connective tissue, and/or the articular disc within the temporomandibular joint.

So the question is, what can cause the increased joint loading, which leads to maladaptation and degenerative changes in the TM joint? Bruxism, clenching, hyperextension, postural compromise, habits related to job or vocation (musicians), and other very repetitive small actions can provide for a robust environment that can result in a cumulative trauma.

Epidemiologic studies reveal a strong association between chronic repetitive forces and the development of osteoarthritis or degenerative joint disease (Buckwalter, 1995). The equation looks like this:

$$\text{Repetition} + \text{Force} + \text{Position} + \text{Time} = \text{Degenerative TM joint disease}$$

Let's consider three applications of this equation:

- Shearing forces on the articular disc at the lateral pole
- Impact of compressive forces on synovial fluid and its protective role in the TM joint
- Secondary inflammatory changes caused by free radical formation

Shearing Forces on the Articular Disc at the Lateral Pole

The attachment of the articular disc to the lateral pole is generally first to become damaged with the resultant anteriomedial disc displacement. The physiologic etiology is unknown, but the anatomy of the articular disc, the shape of the glenoid fossa, and the attachment of the lateral pterygoid provide some interesting insights into the likely confluence of factors contributing to articular disc displacement. The attachment of the articular disc at both the lateral and medial poles is very tenacious and will not easily become torn, stretched, or damaged. It would take a strong force to accomplish this.

During lateral function, the balancing side condyle translates and the working side condyle rotates. In this rotation, because the condyle is not a ball but is elliptical in shape, the lateral pole, which is away from the axis of rotation, actually moves distally. As compressive forces are added to the condyle, such as clenching and shearing forces, force can be generated against the bony lateral lip of the glenoid fossa. This force can stretch or tear the lateral pole attachment during highly repetitive parafunctional movements. When the lateral pole attachment is loosened, the disc is free to move in the direction that the attached muscle (portion of the superior belly of the lateral pterygoid) pulls. This small muscle has about a 15%–20% attachment to the articular disc on the anterior-medial aspect (Loughner et al., 1996). Once the lateral discal attachment is compromised, the disc may be pulled into an anterior-medial direction due to the vectors of force provided by the superior belly of the lateral pterygoid.

Impact of Compressive Forces on Synovial Fluid

The synovial fluid in the TM joint is of utmost importance to the overall function of the articular disc and the coordination of the intricate movement of the mandible. It provides lubrication, nutrition, and oxygen to the tissues of the TM joint, as well as clean-up inside the joint through macrophages that remove debris or other damaging build-up of particles.

Another very important function has been elucidated by Nitzan (1994, 2003). The synovial fluid provides a crucial protective function to the phospholipid layer that provides the slippery ball bearing–like surface of the fibrocartilaginous surface of the articular disc and articular surfaces of the condyle/articular eminence. Normally the articular surfaces are covered with surface-active phospholipids (SAPLs) that are stacked with their hydrophilic end directed toward the articular surface. The hydrophobic end is directed toward the joint space and is bathed in synovial fluid that is rich in hyaluronic acid. If the TM joint is loaded excessively, free radicals are produced in hypoxia reperfusion reactions (see next section). Free radical attack destroys the hyaluronic acid polymers and causes an increase in the viscosity of the synovial fluid to a much more thick or sludgy consistency. The surface active phospholipids are now left unpro tected, allowing the enzyme phospholipase to attack the SAPLs, which results in decreased frictional resistance and damage to the articular surfaces (Nitzan et al., 2001).

Degenerative changes can start small with unraveling of the tightly bound collagen fibrils within the articulating surfaces (fibrillation) and progress to increased matrix degradation, fibrocartilage breakdown, additional synovial fluid alterations (viscosity), impaired function (increased frictional resistance), and incoordination between TM joint components during movement.

Secondary Inflammatory Changes Caused by Free Radical Formation

Free radicals are highly reactive molecules with great tissue-damaging potential. When free radicals are formed they are extremely unstable for as long as they exist, which is not usually very long because they quickly react with nearby molecules that remove the free electron, creating instability in the area. The molecule that absorbs the electron becomes unstable because it is now a free radical with a free electron. So, in a sense, a chain reaction occurs until at least two free radicals react together to form a permanent covalent bond. There are many types of free radicals, but the lipid free radicals are of most importance for our discussion (Milam, 2005).

Free radicals are formed during hypoxia reperfusion reactions. Hypoxia can occur in the TM joint (and muscles) because of compressive forces on the joint. The capsule of the TM joint encloses the whole synovial system, which in fact makes the TM joint a hydraulic system. As compressive forces increase from clenching or other parafunctional activities, the intra-articular pressures rise as high as 220 mm of Hg (Nitzan, 1994). This hydrostatic pressure may exceed the end-capillary perfusion pressure in the TM joint blood vessels (retrodiscal tissue region and other areas). Then as blood flow is reduced, a hypoxia can develop in the synovial tissues (synovial organ), articular tissues, and condylar bone. Intra-articular pressure starting at 9 mm to 17 mmHg has been shown to impede the TM joints' blood supply (Liu and Ho, 1991).

Normal oxygen (O_2) partial pressure in tissue is approximately 21%, but if pressure drops to 5% or 1%, it is not surprising that the rate of cell death (apoptosis) increases (Schneider et al., 2004). As condylar pressure is reduced, blood flow is restored and reperfusion of the cells occurs with renewed supply of oxygen. Milam (2005) elucidated that reperfusion with delivery of oxygen to cell populations previously exposed to hypoxic conditions can lead to an *"explosive production of oxygen derived free radicals"* (italics added).

Lurie et al. (2003) report that hydroxyl ion (OH^-) is the primary free radical formed that attacks the hyaluronic acid in the synovial fluid. Free radicals cannot damage cells or hyaluronic acid unless they exceed the natural antioxidants in the TM joint tissues such as glutathione, superoxide dimutases, and catalases (Regan, Bowler, and Crapo, 2008). Free radicals also attack fibroblasts and chondrocytes. There is evidence that free radicals damage cellular DNA, making DNA less viable to replicate or repair damage in the cartilaginous components of the joint (Grishko et al., 2009). Free radicals attack proteins, lipids, and carbohydrates, damaging synovial fluid, fibrocartilage, cells, and the whole TM joint.

BONY DEGENERATIVE CHANGES

Condylar osseous degenerative changes are strongly correlated with the diagnosis of articular disc displacement. Degenerative joint disease is rare in TM joints with intact, normally positioned articular discs. Normal mandibular condyles appear rounded with a smooth, intact cortical surface. The osseous trabeculation patterns below are directed at an approximately 90-degree angle in a supportive buttressing formation. Once the articular disc is no longer in position or condition to absorb and dissipate the occlusal forces, it should not be surprising that bony degenerative changes develop (Sano et al., 2007).

Degenerative joint disease displays changes on the articular surfaces of the condyle and glenoid fossa of the temporal bone. These changes include flattening of surfaces, irregular surfaces, osteophytic changes, and erosions into the articular surfaces. At onset, the bony changes are small with slight flattening of the articular surface of the condyle.

In the case of progressive, acute degenerative joint disease, during the intermediate stage when the disease is very active, major changes can occur in a one- to two-year window of time. Bony remodeling can occur relatively rapidly through erosive changes with the formation of Ely's cysts below the articular surface. These nonsupportive areas can collapse, resulting in cratering of the load-bearing surface. Osteophytic changes, evidenced radiographically as condylar beaking, are characteristic. The bony trabelculation patterns change, become irregular, and lose their buttressing support arrangement. The condyles lose height and become irregular. Similar changes can occur with the articular eminence becoming much more flattened and irregular. The intermediate breakdown stage is usually noted for pain and crepitus (moderate to coarse).

In the final stages of degenerative joint disease, the condyles become very flattened with an anvil shape. The articular surface is characterized by dense sclerotic bone, which can become smooth (eburnated). The articular eminence is also flattened and sclerotic (de Leeuw et al., 1996; Gruber and Gregg, 2003). The articular space is minimal and the articular disc is often disintegrated. The TM joint may again begin to move more smoothly and even quietly, depending on the quality and quantity of synovial fluid.

GENERAL TREATMENT CONSIDERATIONS

The goals for treating an orthopedic system such as the TM joint and the masticatory system need to address all of the root problems of the contributing factors of orthopedic overload. Occlusal appliances can help relieve some of the excessive forces created through parafunctional activities. Nutritional supplementation can provide antioxidants to help relieve some of the oxidative stress. There are many recent articles discussing the benefit of antioxidants and their value for the health of chondrocytes and benefits for the TM joint (Beecher et al., 2007; Regan, Bowler, and Crapo, 2008). Vitamin C and other antioxidants are likely effective. Vitamin E has not been found to be effective. Reversible treatment modalities need to be applied during painful stages of degenerative joint disease. Multidisciplinary approaches are usually necessary for patients with chronic pain who do not respond to initial level therapy.

SUMMARY

The masticatory system is a dynamic orthopedic system. The masticatory muscles generate forces that are transmitted to all aspects of the system. Under normal loads, these forces provide healthy input to the whole masticatory system, but when the mechanical stress exceeds an individual's adaptive capacity, breakdown occurs. The pathologic changes are expressed in those structures in which that individual is most vulnerable. This vulnerability may be associated with genetics, trauma, systemic factors, or environmental factors. Therefore, dentists, as physicians of the masticatory system, must be able to diagnose and treat the resultant conditions.

REFERENCES

Beecher, B.R., Martin, J.A., Pederson, D.R., et al. (2007). Antioxidants block cyclic loading induced chondrocyte death. *Iowa Orthopaedic Journal*, Vol. 27, pp. 1–8.

Brännström, M. (1966). The hydrodynamics of the dental tubule and pulp fluid: Its significance in relation to dentinal sensitivity. *Annual Meeting of the American Institute of Oral Biology*, Vol. 23, p. 219.

Buckwalter, J.A. (1995). Osteoarthritis and articular cartilage use, disuse, and abuse: Experimental studies. *Journal of Rheumatology*, Vol. 22 (Supplement 43), pp. 13–15.

Cohen, S., Berman, L.H., Blanco, L., et al. (2006). A demographic analysis of root fractures. *Journal of Endodontics*, Vol. 32, pp. 1160–1163.

deBont, L.G. & Stegenga, B. (1993). Pathology of temporomandibular joint internal derangement and osteoarthritis. *International Journal of Oral Maxillofacial Surgery*, Vol. 22, pp. 71–74.

de Leeuw, R., Boering, G., van der Kuijl, B., et al. (1996). Hard and soft tissue imaging of the temporomandibular joint 30 years after diagnosis of osteoarthrosis and internal derangement. *Journal of Oral Maxillofacial Surgery*, Vol. 51, pp. 1270–1280.

Gao, Y.J., Yin, X.M., Wu, H.J. (2001). Relationship between vertical root fracture and the habits of betel nut chewing. *Chinese Dental Journal*, Vol. 26, pp. 161–162.

Grippo, J.O. (1991). Abfractions: A new classification of hard tissue lesions of teeth. *Journal of Esthetic Dentistry*, Vol. 3, pp. 14–19.

Grishko, V.I., Ho, R., Wilson, G.L., et al. (2009). Diminished mitochondrial DNA integrity and repair capacity in OA chondrocytes. *Osteoarthritis and Cartilage*, Vol. 17, pp. 107–113.

Gruber, H.E., and Gregg, J. (2003). Subchondral bone resorption in temporomandibular disorders. *Cells Tissues Organs*, Vol. 174, pp. 17–25.

Hamilton, D. (2008). Functional role of periostin in development and wound repair: Implications for connective tissue disease. *Journal of Cell Communication and Signaling*, Vol. 2, pp. 9–17.

Jafarzadeh, H. (2009). Laser Doppler flowmetry in endodontics: A review. *International Endo Journal*, Vol. 6, pp. 476–490.

Jerge, C.R. (1963). Organization and function of the trigeminal mensencephalic nucleus. *Journal of Neurophysiology*, Vol. 26, pp. 379–392.

Korioth, T.W.P., and Hannam, A.G. (1994). Mandibular forces during simulated clenching. *Journal of Orofacial Pain*, Vol. 8, pp. 178–189.

Kudo, Y., Siriwardena, B.S., Hatano, H., et al. (2007). Periostin: A novel diagnostic and therapeutic target for cancer. *Histology Histopathology*, Vol. 22, pp. 1167–1174.

Kviinnsland, S., Kristiansen, A.B., Kvinnsland, I., et al. (1992). Effect of experimental traumatic occlusion on periodontal and pulpal blood flow. *ACTA Odontalogica Scandinavica*, Vol 50, pp. 211–219.

Liu, S.L., and Ho, T.C. (1991). The role of venous hypertension in the pathogenesis of Legg-Perthes disease: A clinical and experimental study. *Journal of Bone Joint Surgery*, Vol. 73, p. 194.

Loginova, N.K., and Ivanova, E.V. (2008). Masticatory loading influence upon dental pulp functional status and its blood supply. *Stomatologia*, Vol. 87, pp. 13–16.

Loughner, B.A., Gremillon, H.A., Larkin, L.H., et al. (1996). Muscle attachment to the lateral aspect of the articular disc of the human temporomandibular joint. *Oral Surgery, Oral Medicine, Oral Pathololoy, Oral Radiology & Endodontics*, Vol. 82, pp. 139–144.

Lurie, Z., Offer, T., Russo, A., et al. (2003). Do stable nitroxide radicals catalyze or inhibit the degradation of hyaluronic acid? *Free Radical Biology and Medicine*, Vol. 35, pp. 169–178.

Mahan, P.E., Wilkinson, T.M., Gibbs, C.H., et al. (1983). Superior and inferior bellies of the lateral pterygoid muscle EMG activity at basic jaw positions. *Journal of Prosthetic Dentistry*, Vol. 50, p. 710.

Markowitz, K. (1993). Tooth sensitivity mechanisms and management. *Compendium of Continuing Dental Education*, Vol. 14, pp. 1032–1044.

Marting, J.A., et al. (2004). Chondrocyte senescence, joint loading and osteoarthritis. *Clinical Orthopaedics and Related Research*, Vol. 427 (Supplement), pp. 96–103.

Milam, S.B. (2005). Pathogenesis of degenerative temporomandibular joint arthritites. *Odontology*, Vol. 93, pp. 7–15.

Muhlemann, H.R., and Herzog, H. (1961). Occlusal trauma: Effect and impact on the periodontium. *Helv. Odont. Acta*, Vol. 5, pp. 33–39.

Nitzan, D.W. (1994). Intraarticular pressure in the functioning human temporomandibular joint and its alteration by uniform elevation of the occlusal plane. *Journal of Oral Maxillofacial Surgery*, Vol. 51, pp. 671–679.

Nitzan, D.W. (2003). Friction and adhesive forces: Possible underlying causes for temporomandibular joint internal derangement. *Cells Tissues Organs*, Vol. 174, pp. 6–16.

Nitzan, D.W., Nitzan, U., Dan, P., et al. (2001). The role of hyaluronic acid in protecting surface-active phospholipids from lysis by exogenous phospholipase A(2). *Rheumatology*, Vol. 40, pp. 336.

Owens, B.M., and Gallien, G.S. (1995). Noncarious dental "abfraction" lesions in an aging population. *Compendium of Continuing Education in Dentistry*, Vol. 16, pp. 552, 554, 557–558 passim; quiz 562.

Rees, J.S. (2002). The effect of variation in occlusal loading on the development of Abfraction lesions: A finite element study. *Journal Oral Rehabilitation*, Vol. 29, pp. 188–193.

Regan, E.A., Bowler, R.P., and Crapo, J.D. (2008). Joint fluid antioxidants are decreased in osteoarthritic joints compared to joints with macroscopically intact cartilage and subacute injury. *Osteoarthritis Cartilage*, Vol. 16, pp. 515–521.

Rios, H.F., Ma, D., Xie, Y., et al. (2008). Periostin is essential for the integrity and function of the periodontal ligament during occlusal loading in mice. *Journal of Periodontology*, Vol. 79, pp. 1480–1490.

Sano, T., Otonari-Yamamoto, M., Otonari, T., et al. (2007). Osseous abnormalities related to the temporomandibular joint. *Seminars in Ultrasound, CT and MR*, Vol. 28, pp. 213–221.

Sato, S., Tsuchiya, M., Komaki, K., et al. (2009). Synthesis and intracellular transportation of type I precollagen during functional differentiation of odontoblasts. *Histochemistry and Cell Biology*, Vol. 131, pp. 583–591.

Saxton, J.M., Donnelly, A.E., and Roper, H.P. (1994). Indices of free-radical-mediated damage following maximum voluntary eccentric and concentric muscular work. *European Journal of Applied Physiology*, Vol. 8, pp. 189–193.

Schneider, N., Lejeune, J.P., Deby, C., et al. (2004). Viability of equine articular chondrocytes in alginate beads exposed to different oxygen tensions. *The Veterinary Journal*, Vol. 168, pp. 167–173.

Sheikholeslam, A., and Riise, C. (1983). Influence of experimental interfering occlusal contacts on the activity of the anterior temporal and masseter muscles during submaximal and maximal bite in the intercuspal position. *Journal of Oral Rehabilitation*, Vol. 10, pp. 207–214.

Shimizu, N., Ogura, N., Yamaguchi, M., et al. (1992). Stimulation by interleukin-1 of interleukin-6 production by human periodontal ligament cells. *Archives of Oral Biology*, Vol. 37, pp. 743–748.

Sodeyama, T. (1996). Responses of periodontal nerve terminals to experimentally induced occlusal trauma in rat molars: An immunohistochemical study using PGP 9.5 antibody. *Journal of Periodontal Research*, Vol. 31, pp. 235–248.

Vandevska-Radunovic, V., Kristiansen, A.B., Heyeraas, K.J., et al. (1992). Changes in blood circulation in teeth and supporting tissues incident to experimental tooth movement. *Histochemistry*, Vol. 97, pp. 111–120.

Westesson, P.L., and Rohlin, M. (1984). Internal derangement related to osteoarthritis in temporomandibular joint autopsy specimens. *American Journal of Roentgenology*, Vol. 143, pp. 655–660.

Williamson, E.H., and Lundquist, D.O. (1983). Anterior guidance: Its effect on electromyographic activity of the temporal and masseteric muscles. *Journal of Prosthetic Dentistry*, Vol. 49, pp. 816–823.

Yeh, C.J. (1997). Fatigue root fracture: A spontaneous root fracture in nonendodontically treated teeth. *British Dental Journal*, Vol. 182, pp. 261–266.

The Anatomical Basis of Occlusion

Irwin M. Becker, DDS

MANDIBLE POSITION

When examining a dry skull without soft tissue, the observer sees a significant drop in the condylar position during simple hinging, in comparison to the maximum intercuspal position when the teeth are squeezed together. This drop is representative of many shifts that occur when there is not complete harmony between teeth closure and condylar position. During the shift between maximum intercuspation and simple hinging of the mandible, the first point of contact can be clearly observed giving way to full contact. Studies indicate this shift is a natural occurrence in 75% to 85% of any cross-section of the untreated population.

During the early 1980s, investigators started to understand that this drop in condylar position is somehow related to an increase in activity of the muscles of mastication that are directly involved with position of the mandible. The definitive investigation was led by researchers at the University of Florida (Mahan et al., 1983). This study has been very difficult to duplicate as it utilized needle-point electrodes, surgically placed into the bellies of the lateral pterygoid. Not many subjects will volunteer for this kind of dangerous surgery that has the potential of traumatizing the pterygoid plexus of veins and could cause excessive bleeding. While many studies of major, larger muscles utilized surface electrodes, this is one of the only investigations of the opening action of the lateral pterygoid complex. This study found that the action of the two bellies are opposite

Comprehensive Occlusal Concepts in Clinical Practice, by Irwin M. Becker
© 2011 Blackwell Publishing Ltd.

of each other. The inferior belly fires when opening, and the superior is reciprocal, firing when closing.

Another important finding from this landmark investigation was that slight interferences during the centric arc of closure led to increased muscle firing of the entire pterygoid complex. Therefore, any time there is a slide from centric relation arc of closure first point of contact to maximum inter-cuspation, causing a drop in condylar position, there will be concomitant increased muscle activity. In other words, there is an overworking of the pterygoid complex in those patients with an occlusal slide. The lateral pterygoid normally fires when opening but is also called upon to activate during closing if there is a centric relation occlusal interference. A later chapter discusses this as one of the important reasons for occlusal therapy.

USE OF ANTERIOR DEPROGRAMMERS

The above-mentioned phenomenon can be easily demonstrated with any deprogramming device. A patient with a centric relation interference can rest on a deprogramming device for approximately 10 minutes and gain tremendous muscle relaxation. This author routinely utilizes a deprogram-ming device prior to making a centric relation bite registration to ensure more ultimate relaxation of the pterygoid complex. Even when employing the bimanual guidance system described later on, I have found several important advantages of working with the deprogrammer. Both the patient and clinician can feel the difference between normal guidance and guid-ance enhanced with the deprogrammer.

This can be a powerful learning moment for the patient. Often, even during a new patient experience (comprehensive examination)., the patient says, "I wonder if my jaw can feel that relaxed after we are through with treatment?" This can lead to a great conversation and clearly plants a seed of desire to improve one's own occlusal considerations.

The practical benefits of using an anterior deprogrammer follow:

1. Helps in recording centric relation arc of closure
2. Relieves painful and/or tight muscles
3. Helps in identification of occlusal-muscle conditions
4. Increases mandibular movement
5. Could worsen intracapsular derangement

The following references may be consulted to learn more about the repro-ducibility of centric relation and use of a deprogrammer:

1. Lucia, 1964
2. Williamson, 1980
3. Tarantola and Becker, 1997
4. Becker et al., 1999

5. Karl and Foley, 1999
6. Solow, 1999
7. McKee, 2005

PHYSIOLOGIC IMPLICATIONS

The following figure (fig. 4.1). demonstrates the bone-to-bone relationship. The actual hinge takes place between the medial poles of each condyle and medial wall of the glenoid fossa. It is important to observe this simple arc while attempting to duplicate this movement during bimanual guidance.

Early studies (Posselt, 1952) found that once the patient opens more than approximately 10 mm, translation of the mandible begins. Posselt's classic diagram has been further studied in the modern era (Joss and Graf, 1979) by utilizing optoelectronic tracking that is coordinated by an electric camera and an elaborate computer program. These biomechanical movements were later summarized in a classic review in *Dental Clinics of North America* (Weiner, 1995).

When attempting bimanual guidance, the clinician should keep the jaw in simple rotation in the limited arc of closure. Figure 4.2 is an image of the temporomandibular joint, courtesy of French investigator Richard

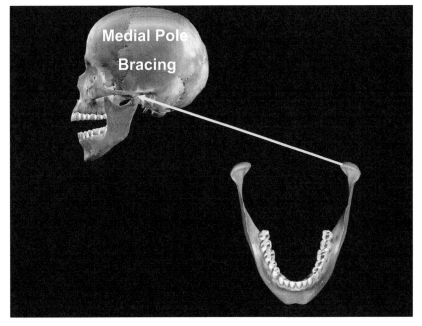

Fig. 4.1. Anatomical relationship in centric relation. © 2010 Wolters Kluwer Health/Lippincott Williams and Wilkins. Reprinted with permission.

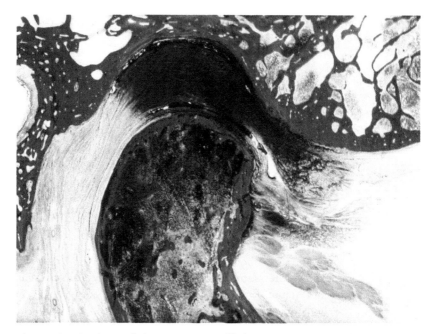

Fig. 4.2. Histology of the temporomandibular joint. Courtesy of Dr. Richard Marguelles-Bonnet.

Margulles-Bonnet. This figure identifies each of the important anatomical parts that come into play during rotation:

- The articulating surface of the condyle
- The two compartments of the articular disc
- The posterior ligament, which tends to hold the disc back like a thick rubber band and prevents more anterior displacement of the disc
- The retro discal tissues that are replete with blood vessels and nerve endings
- The large amount of muscle material anterior to the disc

It was once believed that the tension between the backward pull of the posterior ligament and the forward pull of the superior belly of the lateral pterygoid leads to possible destruction of attachments of the disc, especially when there is sufficient occlusal interferences. It now seems apparent that this is not the case and a balanced equilibrium between these two pulls does exist. Chapter 3 explains the current understanding of discal alteration due to micro-trauma.

One of this author's photographs (fig. 4.3), taken during a Parker Mahan TMJ dissection course, demonstrates the same structures in a fresh cadaver dissection. The condyle disc assembly had just been removed, and Mahan had just cut through the disc, allowing it to butterfly open. This is a clear

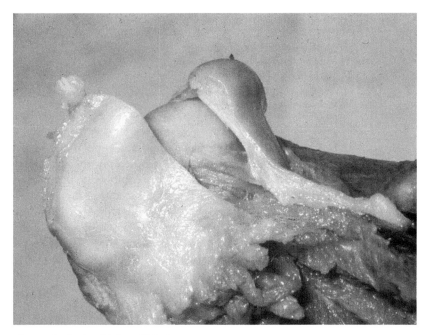

Fig. 4.3. Parker Mahan TMJ dissection.

illustration that only a small percentage of the superior belly actually attaches to the disc and that it happens to be a very weak muscle. It probably acts more like a ligament to simply balance out the tug of the posterior ligament.

Based on these observations and a basic knowledge of the pertinent scientific literature, it is possible to learn techniques that can lead to predictable and repeatable recording of the centric arc of closure.

THE DEFINITION AND REQUIREMENTS OF CENTRIC RELATION

First, a current review of the definition and requirements of centric relation is in order. Please note that if a given patient doesn't meet the requirements outlined in table 4.1, then it would be inappropriate to call his or her position centric relation. It seems that many dentists erroneously attempt to find or record centric on a patient who has a torn disc or eroded medial pole. Alternative descriptions for closure patterns on damaged joints are appropriate to clearly distinguish from the healthy condyle disc assembly. Also, until the patient's mandible can be easily guided into centric, it could be an erroneous recording. It is important to do a complete examination, appropriate diagnostics, and then perform any necessary deprogramming so that a more confident record can be made.

Table 4.1. Definition and requirements of centric relation arc of closure.

(1) Maxillo-mandibular relationship
(2) Healthy condyle-disc assemblies
(3) Seated condyles (superiorly medially)
(4) Muscles unstrained
(5) Comfortable

Dawson and Piper (personal communication, 1985) helped us understand that as long as the medial pole is healthy, the arc can be recorded as centric relation. Therefore, there is a complexity to the timing of one's record that needs to be understood prior to deciding if the record can be considered centric relation. In other words, if there is an indication during the examination that the condyle disc assemblies are damaged or the muscles are tight, or that there is an uncomfortable moment during hinge or loading, then that particular record should be called something other than centric relation. A centric relation record implies a healthy joint and muscle system.

AUTHOR'S PROCEDURE FOR EVALUATING THE JOINTS AND MUSCLES

This author utilizes a specific routine to evaluate the joints and muscles prior to deciding what to call the record. After utilizing the basic exam form shown in chapter 1, the following steps are completed using auscultation (with Doppler) and joint loading with the bimanual guidance technique taught at the Pankey Institute (see table 4.2 for summary).

1. Because joint loading takes place at the medial pole during hinge, the author listens for crepitus during simple arcing of the mandible. If it is quiet, the author assumes an intact medial pole disc assembly. If there is crepitus during simple hinging, the author assumes some damage such as perforation or wrinkling of the disc on or around the medial pole, or some aberration of the actual medial pole from a degenerative or arthritic change.
2. Next, the author listens for crepitus as the patient goes side to side. This time, crepitus indicates alteration of form somewhere other than the medial pole.
3. Then, the author performs the classic light load test to see if there is any discomfort at the 1 to 2 lbs of lifting pressure routinely utilized during the normal bimanual guidance technique. If there is any discomfort during guidance, the author assumes there is some impingement of the retro-discal highly innervated tissues. If there is tenderness on light load, there is no need to go further.

Table 4.2. Evaluation protocol to determine muscle and joint condition.

(1) Crepitus during hinge movement = medial pole alteration
(2) Crepitus during excursive movement = lateral pole alteration
(3) If pain on light load = retro-discal impingement
(4) If pain on heavy load = overworked muscle sprain
(5) If no pain = no real consequence

4. If there is no discomfort, the author tries heavier lifting and loading. The 4 lbs load test is used to investigate if the pterygoid complex is overworked.

By carefully following these steps, the clinician can determine if there is an indication of joint and muscle health or a need to further classify the particular condition. When there is no crepitus and no discomfort, a careful history still needs to be taken in order to rule out past joint pain or joint damage from trauma. In other words, there may be an adapted situation where past disc damage has healed through adaptive fibrotic changes. This is sometimes popularly called a "pseudo disc" and may be totally unresponsive to the light load test. It is the most-often missed diagnostic condition because the clinician is easily fooled if only the load test is utilized. This is why the author always adds the Doppler and records a history during this phase of evaluating the patient's joint condition.

MANDIBLE GUIDANCE TECHNIQUES

It is important to recognize the evolution in techniques utilized to manipulate or guide the mandible toward the centric relation arc of closure. In the 1950s through the mid 1960s, many clinicians applied the push back technique, since most thought the center of rotation of the condyle was rearmost and uppermost in its respective glenoid fossa. This author suffered through this technique being applied to his own jaw with considerable tightness and discomfort during dental school and was so uncomfortable with the experience that the author rejected the concept of centric relation until studying in 1973 with Robert Kaplan, who together with anatomist Harry Sicher opened up a new pathway for thinking about centric relation.

Kaplan espoused the theory that the condyles should be positioned in the uppermost position, based on the anatomy of the fossa (Kaplan, personal communication, 1973). He called this position "the apex of force," which meant the clinician had to stop pushing backward on the chin button (fig. 4.4). Thus, the anterior bite stop that Lucia had been using seemed very helpful (Lucia, 1964).

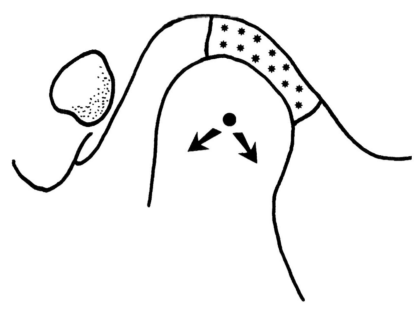

Fig. 4.4. Apex of force diagram. Courtesy of Dr. Robert Kaplan.

In 1974, Dawson began teaching his renowned use of the bimanual technique of guiding the mandible and its condyles into this uppermost position. For many years, the Pankey Institute has utilized both the deprogrammer and the bimanual guidance techniques.

THE BIMANUAL GUIDANCE TECHNIQUE

The bimanual guidance technique requires several specific criteria that, if violated, make the achievement of the seated condyle very unpredictable:

1. The patient's head should be right up against the clinician's gut. This helps stabilize the cranium and also reduces the need to stretch out the clinician's arms, which, when stretched, potentially create a downward vector due to the weight of the arms (fig. 4.5).
2. Next, the arms and shoulders need to be relaxed. Any tension can be perceived by the patient and lead to jaw tightness. The elbows need to be down and in a relaxed position.
3. It is also important to have the dental chair and clinician's chair in proper relationship so the patient's head is at a good supporting height and the clinician's upper legs are parallel to the horizontal.
4. Last, hand and finger position should be specifically aligned as illustrated in figure 4.6. The clinician's little finger and ring finger will

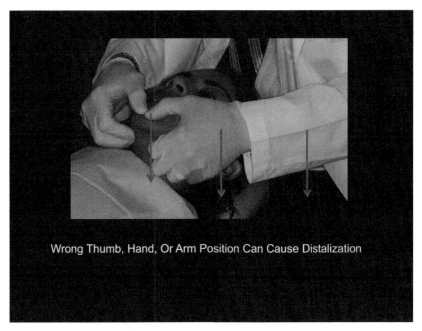

Wrong Thumb, Hand, Or Arm Position Can Cause Distalization

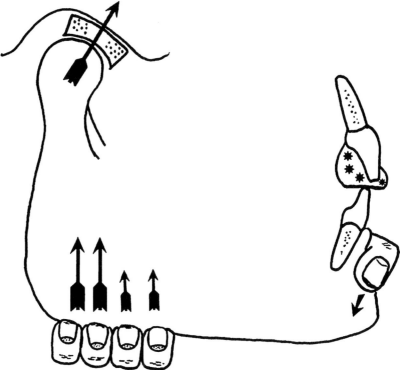

Figs. 4.5 and 4.6. Guidance of the patient's mandible during centric relation arc of closure analysis and/or load testing.

cradle the angle of the mandible. All four fingers will be curled like a "C" onto the inferior osseous border of the mandible. The thumbs will be placed onto the chin button and gently retract the lower lip away from the lower incisal edges to remove any concern of the patient biting the lip.

Doing this also gives the clinician the opportunity to view the incisal edges and gain better understanding of the relationship of the anterior teeth. It is important to observe whether the anterior teeth are coupled (touching) when considering diagnostic workup of the case, including the trial equilibration. The thumb also completes the grasp of the mandible so that the clinician can actually guide and have gentle control of the mandible.

A frequent mistake is to forget to bend the major thumb joint so that it rests on the chin button in a downward direction. Straight thumbs increase the possibility of forcing the mandible rearward.

It is important to sense that all the lifting is coming from the distally placed last two fingers. The others cupped on the inferior border are there simply to gently help grasp the mandible. Thus, these last two small and weak fingers duplicate the direction of the major closing muscles and are then opposed by gentle pressure coming from the downward position of the thumbs. The resultant vector of the condyles is upward with a slight forward cant. This puts the vector going into the clinician's gut.

If all muscles of mastication are relaxed and there are no intracapsular problems, an easy and gentle rotation occurs until the first point of contact. At that point, the clinician can ask the patient to squeeze their teeth together while the clinician envisions the slide for centric relation arc of closure, from first point of contact to full maximum intercuspation. Each time this slide is observed, it is important to remember that one or both condyles are also moving at the same time, most often in some relation to downward or downward and back. From Mahan's work, some degree of muscle activity is expected, mainly in the lateral pterygoid complex.

There may or may not be pain associated with this slide or with gentle manipulation, depending on the condition of the muscles, joints, and associated structures. If everything is normal and healthy, the expectation is there will be no tenderness upon guidance or upon loading at this position. However, if there is pain upon hinge guidance, the pain is likely the result of innervated structures and the discal tissues may have been altered, moved, or perforated.

If muscles are tight or overworked, loading can stretch them, leaving a clinically important burning sensation. In this case, it is important to perform the exercise again after muscle relaxation (therapeutic deprogramming). It is more important to establish the condition and less important to find the actual centric relation arc of rotation during the examination appointment. The author routinely does not find true centric until after bite splint therapy.

FUNCTIONAL AND PARAFUNCTIONAL MOVEMENTS

It is critical to the implementation of material imparted in this text to differentiate between functional and parafunctional movements of the masticatory system. Function is obvious during masticating, swallowing, or doing any usual and ordinary activity of the cranio-mandibular system and its associated structures. Parafunction occurs when no real purpose is being achieved other than putting the mandible in an otherwise harmful or bizarre position. Often this is repeated and held for long periods of time. It can become an adapted habit if not developed into a destructive pattern. As stated earlier, the patient usually is unaware of when they do this activity.

The literature is replete with definitions and examples of parafunction, but very few studies describe the actual cause of parafunction. In 1987, Moss et al. found some degree of predictability between EMG analyses and parafunctional clenching and bruxing movements. In 1980, Silvestri described the differences between the muscle physiology of functional activities of chewing and the parafunctional habits of clenching and bruxing. Thus, for many years now, researchers have understood that even at the cellular level there is a difference in parafunctional activity.

Near the same time, Okeson described parafunction as an interaction of occlusal interferences and psychological related stress. He emphasized that the actual causative factors must be identified in order to best treat the problem of parafunctional activity. All these years later, it remains unclear if the clinician can actually stop parafunction. It is the basis of this text that the clinician has the best opportunity to reduce the effects of parafunction by reducing the hyper muscle activity associated with parafunctional activity. Therefore, the clinician will be most attracted to the chapters dedicated to bite splint therapy and establishing a physiologic occlusion, not to stop parafunction but to make it a less destructive habit by application of physiologic occlusion.

This author's understanding of excursive movements and excursive interferences is based on the groundbreaking work of Belser and Hannam (1985). These researchers found that removal of excursive interferences leads to a canine guidance that greatly reduces the muscle activity of the major elevator muscles. It is noteworthy that in their study, canine protected occlusions did not alter muscle activity during normal mastication; however, muscle activity was significantly reduced during parafunctional activity. Nonworking (balancing) interferences led not only to greatly increased closing muscle activity but also altered the distribution of muscle activity during parafunctional clenching. They postulated that this redistribution might affect the nature of reaction forces at the temporomandibular joints. Therefore, when considering the role of micro-trauma as discussed in chapter 3, consider that this increased muscle activity during parafunction can be harmful to teeth, joints, and all associated structures. This is the strongest scientific rationale for organizing occlusions to help reduce potentially damaging muscle activity. It would be a good habit to read and study every project concerning muscle physiology that is written by Alan Hannam.

Baba offered another series of papers that also demonstrated that patients, who had artificially created balancing side interferences, had increased activity in the temporal muscles. However, this study (Baba, 1991) did not seem to distinguish parafunctional behavior from patient-directed maximum clenching. It is possible that a given patient may not be able to simulate actual parafunctional activity on command.

Kampe (1987) observed more signs and symptoms of wear, muscle tenderness to palpation, headache, tiredness during mastication, and joint sounds in restored dentitions than in intact dentitions. This author would have preferred to have these restored dentitions evaluated for the presence of centric and eccentric interferences.

In an evaluation of patients with nocturnal bruxism, Attanasio (1991) noted that many patients find a degree of adaptation. This study found that in some individuals the capacity of adaptation will be exceeded by the cumulative forces of this parafunctional behavior resulting in pain and dysfunction of the masticatory system. His article discusses the history, nature, possible causes, and effects of bruxism.

Wood (1987) presents a wonderful review of masticatory muscle function, suggesting that eventually clinicians will be able to predict, after careful observation and analysis, when there is increased muscle activity. In Wood's study, clenching and increased tooth contacts during excursive movements all led to increased muscle activity.

An interesting study by Harper, de Bruin, and Burcea (1997) on pre- and postorthognathic surgery patients who had retrognathic mandibles showed that these patients had different muscle recruitment patterns than normal subjects, and after surgery there was adaptation in the phasic timing of jaw muscle activity. This type of study is not meant to indicate that all patients should be treated as Class 1 status. Rather, that anyone with increased posterior contacts in excursive movement has predictably increased muscle recruitment.

In a critically important paper, Israel (1999) studied the relationship between parafunctional masticatory activity and arthroscopically diagnosed temporomandibular joint pathology. This study intended to assess the hypothesis that the presence of parafunctional activity leads to increased arthroscopically diagnosed pathology. It was concluded that parafunctional masticatory activity and its influence on joint loading contribute to osteoarthritis of the temporomandibular joint. Such osteoarthritis is associated with adhesions of the joint. Because of the many potential routes of damage to the joint from overload of the system during parafunctional activity, clinicians must identify and address parafunction during nonsurgical, surgical, and postsurgical treatment regimens. This text very much agrees with these and other conclusions from many studies and empirical observations that implicate parafunction as a major culprit in pathological end points of the cranio-mandibular system.

LOCATION OF CONDYLE LOADING

Figures 4.7 and 4.8 illustrate that loading takes place at the medial pole when hinging. However, as soon as the act of translation begins, the load starts to move away from the medial pole and onto some aspect on top or

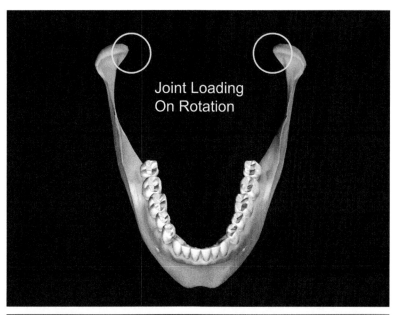

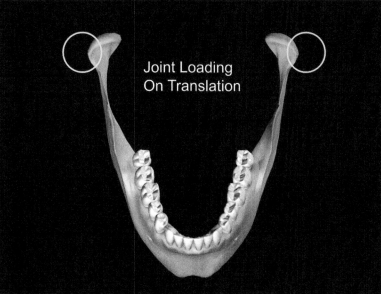

Figs. 4.7 and 4.8. Guidance of the patient's mandible during centric relation arc of closure analysis and/or load testing. © 2010 Wolters Kluwer Health/Lippincott Williams and Wilkins. Reprinted with permission.

toward the lateral pole. This phenomenon can be helpful in determining the condition of the disc and the extent of damage, as well as the progression of the damage. This can be extremely important in view of the history the patient presents. From a clinical examination perspective, the condition cannot be precisely determined without MRI imaging; however, a general indication of the severity or relative mildness of the joint condition can be determined. Work by Piper (personal communication, 1990) indicates that most joint breakdown begins at the lateral pole, and if it does continue, it works itself more toward the medial pole. Thus, crepitus heard on rotation signifies a worsened condition, whereas crepitus on excursive movement indicates a typically less threatening condition.

Because of the nature of the change in loading and because of the variations found in a particular part of the joint, there may be some patients who are susceptible to joint problems. Sometimes there is a larger, more prominent lateral rim to the glenoid fossa. Those patients with this anomaly may be prone to lateral pole defects in the disc simply because the lateral rim begins to act as a boney interference and partially entraps the lateral aspects of the disc at an early age. If the patient has any tendency to move out laterally to the point where damage occurs, there is a much greater susceptibility.

This author feels it is important to simply identify those patients with severe joint conditions that manifest themselves with medial pole pathologies. These cases have joint crepitus during simple hinge movement, whereas crepitus upon lateral movements indicate a more generalized and a less serious breakdown of structures. As long as there appears to be a healthy medial pole, the clinician can describe the joint condition when seated as centric relation or at least an adapted centric position. It is critical to add a history to this part of the exam, as there might have been damage years ago and now scar tissue might have eliminated or masked some of the signs upon loading.

THE ENVELOPE OF PARAFUNCTION

A consistent observation of when and where pathological wear has been manifested actually caused this author to commit to writing this text. It has become obvious that wear essentially occurs because of parafunctional activity. This author doesn't believe that wear occurs during normal function of chewing or swallowing.

For many years, signs of wear were considered indicative of the normal chewing function, and this author was intently careful to create restorative inclines that would not invade or violate the patient's acquired envelope of function (also called the "envelope of movement" or "chewing stroke"). Chapter 5 will address this issue in great detail.

In recent years, the author has taken a slightly different approach. Patterns of wear are no longer viewed as the envelope of function. Patterns of anterior and/or posterior wear are all believed to come from parafunctional activity. When attempting to create a predictable and long-lasting new guidance pattern, the author generally tries to match the type of parafunctional wear patterns. To determine if the patient can tolerate a longer, steeper guidance for esthetic reasons, a composite mock-up or provisional is worn for a longer trial period. Even though wear patterns are viewed as parafunctional symptoms, the author evaluates violations of the envelope of function for comfort and chewing considerations.

THE IMPORTANCE OF TIMING OF THE SEATED CONDYLE DISC ASSEMBLY

If the clinician attempts to seat the condyle prior to proper positioning of the disc, there could be resulting impingement of sensitive retro-discal tissues. If there is an attempt to seat the condyle prior to muscle relaxation, there could be a burning sensation coming from the overworked lateral pterygoid complex of muscles. The author believes clinicians are sometimes disappointed in the results of working with centric relation because they miss the importance of its timing. As long as the medial pole is in place, the clinician should be able to achieve comfortable seating. As mentioned before, it is important to do an exam so that the clinician has a reasonable impression about the condition of the disc. Certainly, if there are degenerative or arthritic conditions, full seating may need to be put off until some resolution is obtained.

This resolution may simply be maintenance of a longer-term occlusal bite splint. Often this transitional bite splint needs to be adjusted differently than in the case of a healthy joint. The clinician may need to adjust it to the patient's own comfortable closure and not guide it into the seated position. The astute clinician figures this out because either it was uncomfortable to adjust toward seating or the results were simply not rewarding for the patient or clinician.

Ultimately, comfort is the guide in deciding when to change from using the patient's own closure to using the guided adjustment. Almost always, the clinician hopes to get to a seated position, but only when the disc assembly is in place can it be called centric relation. Otherwise, the clinician may have to settle for a treatment position that the joint condition dictates.

Once intracapsular abnormalities are found, the decision tree becomes more complicated and generally takes more time. With common sense and awareness of any abnormality in the involved structures, the clinician can bring some predictability to managing these more difficult and challenging diagnostic problems. It may be an oversimplification, but this author has observed that most patients are eventually well enough to move ahead with conventional bite splint therapy that leads to guided adjustment.

Some need to first go through a period of healing with their own comfortable closure.

REFERENCES

Attanasio, R. (1991). Nocturnal bruxism and its clinical arrangement. *Dental Clinics of North America*, Vol. 35, pp. 245–252.

Baba, K. (1991). Influences of balancing-side interference on jaw function. *Kokubyo Gakkai Zasshi*, Vol. 58, pp. 118–137.

Belser, U.C., and Hannam, A.G. (1985). The influence of altered working-side occlusal guidance on masticatory muscles and related jaw movement. *Journal of Prosthetic Dentistry*, Vol. 53, pp. 406–413.

Harper, R.P., de Bruin, H., and Burcea, I. (1997). Muscle activity during mandibular movements in normal and mandibular retrognathic subjects. *Journal of Oral Maxillofacial Surgery*, Vol. 55, pp. 225–233.

Israel, H. (1999). The use of arthroscopic surgery for treatment of temporomandibular joint disorders. *Journal of Oral Maxillofacial Surgery*, Vol. 57, pp. 579–582.

Joss, A., and Graf, H. (1979). A method for analysis of human mandibular occlusal movement. *SSO Schweiz Monatsschr Zahnheilkd*, Vol. 89, pp. 1211–1220.

Kampe, T. (1987). Function and dysfunction of the masticatory system in individuals with intact and restored dentitions: A clinical, psychological and physiological study. *Swedish Dental Journal Supplement*, Vol. 42, pp. 1–68.

Lucia, V.O. (1964). A technique for recording centric relation. *Journal of Prosthetic Dentistry*, Vol. 14, pp. 492–505.

Mahan, P.E., Wilkinson, T.M., Gibbs, C.H., et al. (1983). Superior and inferior bellies of the lateral pterygoid muscle EMG activity at basic jaw positions. *Journal of Prosthetic Dentistry*, Vol. 50, pp. 710–718.

Moss, R.A., Villarosa, G.A., Cooley, J.E., et al. (1987). Masticatory muscle activity as a function of parafunctional, active and passive oral behavioral patterns. *Journal of Oral Rehabilitation*, Vol. 14, pp. 361–370.

Okeson, J.P. (1981). *Etiology* and treatment of occlusal pathosis and associated facial pain. *Journal of Prosthetic Dentistry*, Vol. 45, pp. 199–204.

Posselt, U. (1952). Studies in the mobility of the mandible. *Acta Odontologica Scandinavica*, Vol. 10 (Supplement), pp. 1–160.

Silvestri, A.R. Jr, Cohen, S.N., Connolly, R.J. (1980). Muscle physiology during functional activities and parafunctional habits. *Journal of Prosthetic Dentistry*, Vol. 44, pp. 64–67.

Weiner, S.W. (1995). Biomechanics of occlusion and the articulator. *Dental Clinics of North America*, Vol. 39, pp. 257–284.

Wood, W.W. (1987). A review of masticatory muscle function. *Journal of Prosthetic Dentistry*, Vol. 57, pp. 222–223.

ADDITIONAL RECOMMENDED READING

Buyle-Bodin, Y., Lund, T.M., and Robinson, P.J. (1986). Canine slope and glenoid cavity morphology: Relationships with dental wear. *Journal of Prosthetic Dentistry*, Vol. 56, pp. 312–317.

Clark, G.T., et al. (1999). Sixty-eight years of experimental occlusal interference studies: What have we learned? *Journal of Prosthetic Dentistry*, Vol. 82, pp. 704–713.

Coffey, J.P., et al. (1989). A preliminary study of the effects of tooth guidance on the working-side condylar movement. *Journal of Prosthetic Dentistry*, Vol. 62, pp. 157–162.

D'Amico, A. (1962). Functional occlusion of the natural teeth of man. *Journal of Prosthetic Dentistry*, Vol. 11, pp. 899–915.

deBont, L.G.M., et al. (1986). Osteoarthritis and internal derangement of the temporomandibular joint: A light microscope study. *Journal of Oral Maxillofacial Surgery*, Vol. 44, pp. 634–643.

Forsberg, C.M., Eliasson, S., and Westergren, H. (1991). Face height and tooth eruption in adults: A 20-year follow-up investigation. *European Journal of Orthodontics*, Vol. 13, pp. 249–254.

Geering, A.H. (1974). Occlusal interferences and functional disturbances of the masticatory system. *Journal of Clinical Periodontology*, Vol. 1, pp. 112–119.

Granados, J.I. (1979). The influence of the loss of teeth and attrition on the articular eminence. *Journal of Prosthetic Dentistry*, Vol. 42, pp. 78–85.

Israel, H.A., et al. (1999). The relationship between parafunctional masticatory activity and arthroscopically diagnosed temporomandibular joint pathology. *Journal of Oral Maxillofacial Surgery*, Vol. 57, pp. 1034–1039.

Ito, T., et al. Loading on the temporomandibular joints with five occlusal conditions. *Journal of Prosthetic Dentistry*, Vol. 56, pp. 478–484.

Lytle, J.D. (1990). The clinician's index of occlusal disease: Definition, recognition, and management. *International Journal of Periodontal Restorative Dentistry*, Vol. 10, pp. 103–124.

Lytle, J.D. (2001). Occlusal disease revisited: Part I. Function and parafunction. *International Journal of Periodontal Restorative Dentistry*, Vol. 21, pp. 265–271.

Lytle, J.D. (2001). Occlusal disease revisited: Part II. *International Journal of Periodontal Restorative Dentistry*, Vol. 21, pp. 273–279.

Moffett, B.C., et al. (1964). Articular remodeling in the adult human temporomandibular joint. *American Journal of Anatomy*, Vol. 115, pp. 119–142.

Mongini, F. (1972). Remodelling of the mandibular condyle in the adult and its relationship to the condition of the dental arches. *Acta Anatomica*, Vol. 822, pp. 437–453.

Mongini, F. (1980). Condylar remodeling after occlusal therapy. *Journal of Prosthetic Dentistry*, Vol. 43, pp. 568–577.

Nickerson, J.W., and Boering, G. (1989). Natural course of osteoarthrosis as it relates to internal derangement of the temporomandibular joint. *Oral Maxillofacial Surgery Clinics of North America*, Vol. 1, pp. 27–45.

Nitzan, D.W. (1994). Intraarticular pressure in the functioning human temporomandibular joint and its alteration by uniform elevation of the occlusal plane. *Journal of Oral Maxillofacial Surgery*, Vol. 52, pp. 671–679.

Nitzan, D.W. (1997). The "anchored disc phenomenon": A proposed etiology for sudden-onset, severe, and persistent closed lock of the temporomandibular joint. *Journal of Oral Maxillofacial Surgery*, Vol. 55, pp. 797–802.

Nitzan, D.W. (2001). The process of lubrication impairment and its involvement in temporomandibular joint disc displacement: A theoretical concept. *Journal of Oral Maxillofacial Surgery*, Vol. 59, pp. 36–45.

Oberg, T., Carlsson, G.E., and Fagers, C.M. The temporomandibular joint. A morphologic study on a human autopsy. *Acta Odontologica Scandinavica*, Vol. 29, pp. 349–384.

Ratcliff, S., Becker, I.M., and Quinn L. (2001). Type and incidence of cracks in posterior teeth. *Journal of Prosthetic Dentistry*, Vol. 86, pp. 168–172.

Schellhas, K.P. (1989). Unstable occlusion and temporomandibular joint disease. *Journal of Clinical Orthodontics*, Vol. 23, pp. 322–327.

Schellhas, K.P., Piper, M.A., and Omlie, M.R. (1990). Facial skeleton remodeling due to temporomandibular joint degeneration: An imaging study of 100 patients. *American Journal of Neuroradiology*, Vol. 11, pp. 541–551.

Siebert, G. (1981). Recent results concerning physiological tooth movement and anterior guidance. *Journal of Oral Rehabilitation*, Vol. 8, pp. 479–493.

Standlee, J.P., Caput, A.A., and Ralph, J.P. (1979). Stress transfer to the mandible during anterior guidance and group function eccentric movements. *Journal of Prosthetic Dentistry*, Vol. 41, pp. 35–39.

Stegenga, B. (2000). Osteoarthritis of the temporomandibular joint organ and its relationship to disc displacement. *Journal of Orofacial Pain*, Vol. 15, pp. 193–205.

Zarb, G.A., and Carlssson, G.E. (1999). Temporomandibular disorders: Osteoarthritis. *Journal of Orofacial Pain*, Vol. 13, pp. 295–306.

Accepted Occlusal Principles Involved in Physiologic Occlusion

Irwin M. Becker, DDS

ANTERIOR GUIDANCE AND ITS ROLE IN EVERYDAY DENTISTRY

Selecting the appropriate teeth to guide the mandible in all excursive movements is something practitioners might do on a daily basis. Typically, the correct choice is the anterior-most set of teeth that are in position and are healthy and stable enough to take the load of guidance. We no longer call this "incisal guidance" or "canine guidance."

There are essentially three basic requirements of anterior selected teeth that will serve as appropriate guidance. (1) They should disclude the rest of the posterior teeth in all excursive movements, and (2) they should do so smoothly, so that there are no catches, hang-ups, or rapid drop-off from these teeth to others that will take over, once the jaw moves far enough into a parafunctional position. (3) They should be able to match precisely in an edge-to-edge position, whether in straight protrusive or in lateral guidance in a cuspid edge-to-edge position.

Figures 5.1 through 5.3 demonstrate this hand-off occurring right at the cuspid-to-cuspid position as the lower lingual angle crosses over the labial angle of the maxillary cuspid. However, as soon as the two teeth line up over each other, there should be enough of a flat landing area to stabilize this position. Critical to this movement are the leading and trailing edges or bevels that lead up to and follow the actual edge-to-edge positions.

Comprehensive Occlusal Concepts in Clinical Practice, by Irwin M. Becker
© 2011 Blackwell Publishing Ltd.

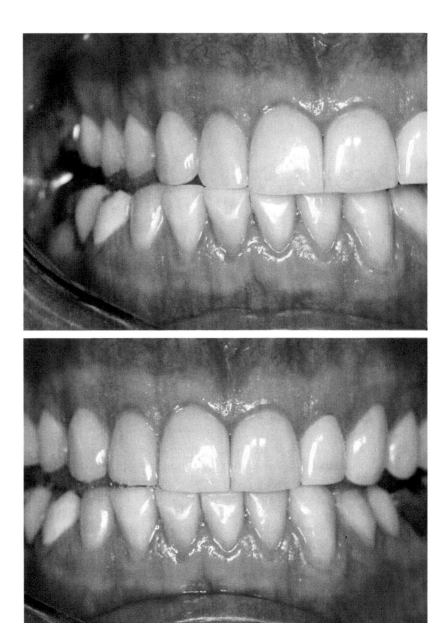

Figs. 5.1–5.3. Crossover details.

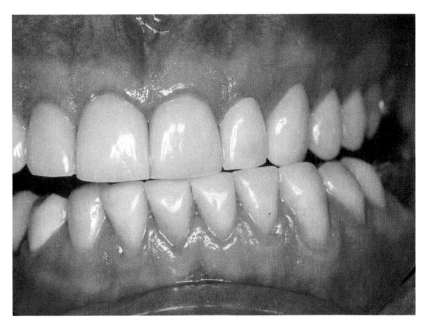

Figs. 5.1–5.3. *Continued*

In protrusive, a similar phenomenon occurs. Lower incisal line angles in front and behind the pitch or flat landing areas of the incisors make the potential movements occur smoothly. Therefore, moving on to the edge-to-edge position not only feels stable, but creates a braced position for the patient. Also, when the patient slides around on the edges, the movement is smooth.

The question remains, Which teeth are appropriate for guidance? In straight protrusive, the author normally selects the two maxillary central incisors and the lower two central incisors. But this requires that the selected teeth be healthy, periodontally strong, and in reasonably good position. Otherwise, the contact to all four incisors may have to be broadened. The selection of guidance teeth very much depends on periodontal condition, tooth structure condition, and tooth position. Leaving a guidance surface in dentin would likely result in lack of stability.

Figures 5.4 and 5.5 demonstrate the typical tracking that occurs along the marginal ridges of the upper incisors and smoothly transfers to the actual incisal edge. A flat pitch to the edge and rounded soft bevels leading up to that edge-to-edge surface are preferable. Not only is anterior guidance discluded, but the remaining posterior teeth immediately disclude in a smooth fashion.

The phonetics and esthetics could be affected by these changes. So it is important that achieving esthetic harmony is also a requirement of appropriate guidance. It is commonly understood that the trial workup is a best

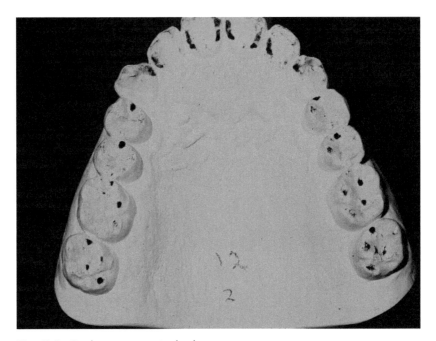

Fig. 5.4. Guidance on marginal ridges.

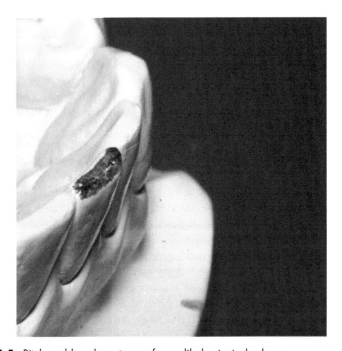

Fig. 5.5. Pitch and bevel anatomy of mandibular incisal edges.

guess and that phonetic and esthetic acceptability need to be evaluated in the mouth through provisional restorations or bonded composite mock-ups.

A checklist for this evaluation can be very helpful:

- Wear
- Mobility changes
- Breakage
- Decementation
- Discomfort
- Phonetic changes
- Esthetic acceptability

There is sufficient literature indicating the science of the relationship between posterior excursive interferences and increased muscle activity during bruxing. The powerful closing muscles are predictably affected whenever immediate posterior disclusion is not achieved. Hannam et al. (1977), Manns et al. (1979, 1981, 1987), Williamson and Lundquist (1983), and Riise and Sheikholeslam (1982) are a few of the classic researchers who have proven that this phenomenon takes place. Therefore, it is critical in every form of dentistry, whether in natural occlusion, restored occlusion, or bite splint therapy, that the universal goal of posterior disclusion be achieved.

Figures 5.6 through 5.8 demonstrate the muscles involved. Chapter 6 will further elaborate. It is important to remember that overactive muscles may or may not be painful. A sign of their hyperactivity might only appear when carefully palpating these muscles and comparing one side to the other.

EXCEPTIONS AND COMPROMISES

Sometimes, when the upper cuspids are either missing or out of position or periodontally weakened, one cannot utilize them reasonably for lateral guidance. The upper first bicuspid must then be used as a crutch. Therefore, a form of group function is called upon in such compromises. Perhaps the patient declined orthodontics and/or orthognathic surgery. Both bicuspids may have to be used to initiate the lateral movement and then switched over to cuspids and/or incisors as soon as reasonable in the act of moving laterally.

In other words, every patient does not have to be in cuspid Class 1 arrangement. However, one must be very careful in selecting bicuspids to start the movement, for the following reasons: (1) These posterior teeth have the capacity to fire up those closing muscles. (2) If they are already worn, they may not be stable for the long term. (3) The ability to have them shift toward the anterior teeth smoothly must be in the mind of the

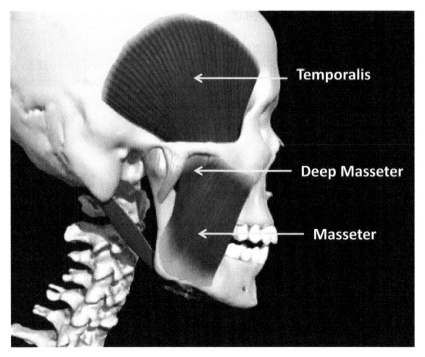

Fig. 5.6. Temporalis and masseter muscles (elevators). © 2010 Wolters Kluwer Health/Lippincott Williams and Wilkins. Reprinted with permission.

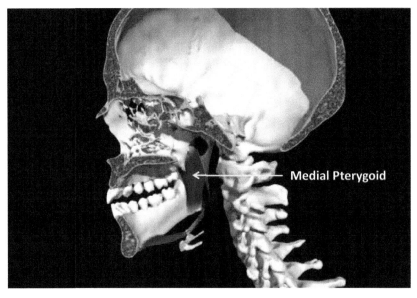

Fig. 5.7. Medial pterygoid muscle (elevator). © 2010 Wolters Kluwer Health/Lippincott Williams and Wilkins. Reprinted with permission.

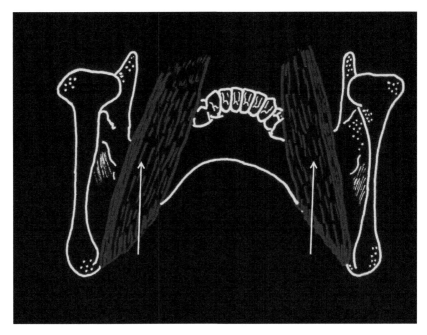

Fig. 5.8. Medial pterygoid—contributes greatly to the vertical loading.

clinician. Rubber wheel detailing out of this progressive guidance from bicuspid to incisor is one of the most difficult adjustments. Another thing to note is that once one has achieved good centric stops, this progressive guidance must not interfere or remove any of the critically important centric stops. Chapter 10 further explains this issue.

A level occlusal and incisal plane makes it much easier to correct the guidance system. When a lower cuspid is sticking up above the normal plane of occlusion, it often is misperceived as interference in protrusive against the upper lateral incisal embrasure. This author observes that a dentist reaches one level of maturation when he or she realizes the need to correct a supererupted upper molar in order to correctly restore a lower crown, bridge, or implant. The next big maturation occurs when the dentist realizes that in order to restore upper anterior teeth he or she may need to first correct the irregular or inclined incisal plane. This observation will be stressed again in this text.

NEGATIVE EFFECTS OF DISTALIZING INCLINES

Even though the orthodontic literature claims that Class 2 occlusions do not exhibit any increased risk, the author believes that the potential of guidance placed on the distal slope of maxillary cuspids or even bicuspids could result in posterior directed forces, thus adding undue stress on the condyle disc assembly. It would have to be combined with some parafunctional activity to perpetuate a serious threat. That being said, it is suggested that one should attempt to decrease the steepness of any distalizing incline. This could be especially beneficial in compromised group function cases or almost any Class 2 case. The bottom line in this particular discussion is (1) to preferably have the guidance situated down the middle or anterior aspect of the upper canines and (2) to observe any previous wear patterns or other sign of occlusal instability in these same situations.

CENTRIC STABILITY

The Pankey Institute has been a longtime proponent of a freedom in centric style morphology. Figure 5.9 demonstrates that a simple, predictable, and practical type of occlusion has the centric holding cusp tips hitting on flat opposing landing areas called the centrum. Usually about 0.5 mm. wide, this type of contact is nondirective, with no incline able to shift the mandible and condyle. The author has noticed much greater long-term stability in this kind of occlusal scheme, especially when compared to the tripod type of contact.

Figure 5.10 illustrates the older gnathological style that requires a fully adjustable articulator to prepare grooves and sluice ways for the centric

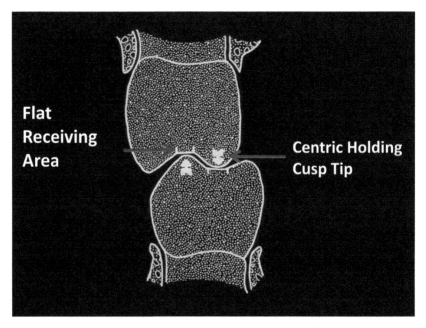

Fig. 5.9. Freedom in and out of centric morphology (cusp to flat receiving area).

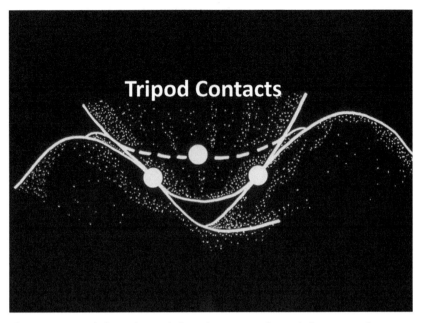

Fig. 5.10. Gnathological morphology (more natural morphology—tripod contacts cusp tip into fossa).

holding cusp tip to freely escape. Today, many dentists make use of the centrum concept, not only because it is practical but also because they have found greater long-term stability. This author has observed as years go by and teeth, joints, and associated cranio-mandibular structures change slightly, many tripoded cases begin to hit only on incline contacts, whereas occlusal schemes involving cusp tips hitting flat landing areas are still hitting on the flat areas. Thus, maintenance over, say, a 10-year period may only require a slight rubber wheel touch-up.

The author has found that tripoded cases need constant re-equilibration and thus believes the very best opportunity for long-term stability of occlusal forces is to have simultaneous contacts on all posterior well-formed cusp tips hitting on flat receiving areas so that the forces are directed along the long axis of each well-positioned tooth.

PLACEMENT OF CONTACTS

Figures 5.11 and 5.12 demonstrate appropriate, potential occlusal contacts. Note that they can be almost anywhere on each tooth as long as they are parallel to the long axis. Marginal ridge areas make good locations, as do the transverse ridges of upper molars. Only rarely can one achieve a nice flat contact down into the central groove areas of maxillary or mandibular

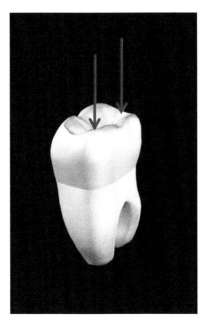

Fig. 5.11. Potential mandibular flat receiving areas. © 2010 Wolters Kluwer Health/Lippincott Williams and Wilkins. Reprinted with permission.

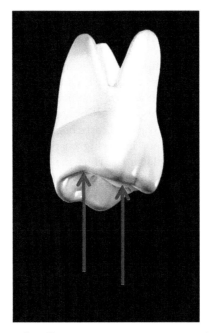

Fig. 5.12. Potential maxillary flat receiving areas. © 2010 Wolters Kluwer Health/Lippincott Williams and Wilkins. Reprinted with permission.

molars. Whereas they would make good locations for tripod contacts, the opposing cusp tip is usually not long enough to bottom out onto a centrum. The key is to have these locations stable and also designed such that with just a basic understanding of anatomy and ridge and groove direction, one can obtain an immediate disclusion.

FREEDOM IN AND OUT OF CENTRIC

The principle of freedom emerged and evolved out of the centric proposition of the 1950s. Back then, an objective of the Pankey Mann Schuyler methodology was to make sure occlusal contacts occurred on large, flat surfaces that extended from maximum intercuspal position to the retruded contact. Since the anatomical basis of centric relation had not yet been determined, practitioners, in order to be safe and not have any deflective inclines, flattened all possible contact out from the two extreme popular opinions of the day.

As dentists began to accept the superior positioned condylar placement, long centric was no longer needed. Interestingly, the author has observed many long-standing cases that remained stable for over half a century based on long centric. So it did work and can last.

Today we have a much better understanding of the condylar starting point, as well as the need for appropriate anterior guidance to create immediate posterior.

There are really two parts to the concept of freedom in centric. First is the aforementioned centrum landing area. This is part of freedom as there are no potential inclines to force the closure to slide. There are no inclines to drag as soon as the mandible goes into excursion. Secondly, the anterior teeth must not hit harder than any posterior contact. If they do hit harder, the possibility exists for distalizing inclines occurring on anterior teeth, actual migration, spreading apart, and even wear patterns.

The author makes it a point after any occlusal adjustment, be it bite splint therapy, natural occlusion, or restored dentition, to always do the following protocol.

1. As the patient sits up and leans forward slightly, ask the patient how the front teeth feel when they tap-tap.
2. Place your fingers across the upper anterior teeth and ask the patient to tap again, feeling for any fremitus. This potential palpable movement manifests when anterior teeth hit harder than posterior contact.
3. Mark the teeth again when the patient is sitting up and slightly leaning forward.
4. Gently reduce down any contact that produces fremitus. Most patients actually feel better when the anterior teeth are just lightly touching. The anterior teeth should touch slightly less than the firm posterior contact, but there should still be contact.

The posterior contacts are for hard centric stops. They have the power to stop vertical closure, so they are similar to offensive linemen. The anterior contacts are similar to ballet dancers. Even though they are strong, they are very light on their feet. They touch lightly and are prepared to do their gliding and guiding.

Previously mentioned studies indicate that when there are no slides from first point of contact to maximum intercuspal contact, the lateral pterygoid complex reaches its normal muscle input. The intention of achieving no slide from light closure to hard closure reflects this understanding of muscle recruitment. The most stable and neuromuscular-relaxed condition occurs when all teeth touch simultaneously (anterior teeth touching slightly less) and there are no deflections due to incline contacts. This, coupled with an anterior guidance that is appropriate for the particular case at hand, provides predictable stability for the long haul.

Figure 5.13 likely indicates the most important schematic for understanding posterior occlusion. Each clinician would do well to memorize and understand the classic potential movements of cusp tips across their opposing anatomy. These pathways explain the basic anatomy, as well as the requisite grooves and pathways that enable immediate posterior disclusion. This set of diagrams is from Dr. Henry Tanner (1982, personal

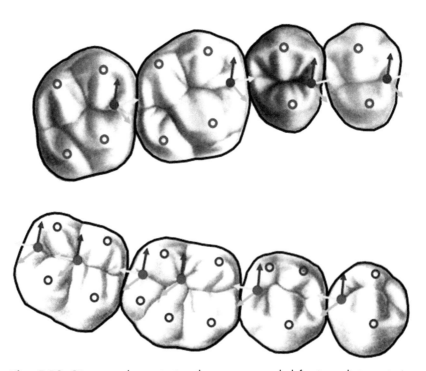

Fig. 5.13. Diagrams demonstrating the grooves needed for immediate posterior disclusion out of the flat receiving areas.

communication) and is perhaps his greatest gift to dentistry. Once you have these diagrams memorized, you will have an easier time with your direct carvings, as well as adjustment of natural and restored dentitions.

THE POWER WIGGLE

One other aspect of occlusion is to evaluate the effect that certain patients have when either clenching or bruxing in an abbreviated movement. They do not move laterally much at all but rather appear to widen their contact on the flat area provided. This is observed sometimes on both bite splint adjustments and natural dentitions.

It could be a result of lack of immediate anterior guidance. It also could be an example of the potential movement or flexure of the mandible. Another explanation is a slight incline on one or more of the centrum receiving areas. After clearing out all the above-mentioned possibilities, the astute clinician realizes that this patient may need slightly more freedom and end up with a wider centrum.

The dentists may need to refine over and over these contacts until the patient regains some comfort and has once again established immediate posterior disclusion. When using both black ribbons for centric and red for eccentric, the best that one can end up with is no red outside the black landing pad. Typically that results in the longest stable situation possible for the power wiggle patient.

REORGANIZING OCCLUSIONS FOR BOTH FUNCTION AND ESTHETICS

This author believes there is an appropriate order in which to consider reorganizing a patient's occlusion. With all that has been presented in this text, there remains an array of choices from which the comprehensive dentist can choose. The clinician may want to evaluate the following list of options based on degree of invasiveness. Most often, the clinician chooses the least invasive treatment that accomplishes the desired endpoint of therapy. The following list begins with the least invasive and ends with most complex and invasive, therefore ending with the most difficulty, greatest risk, and clearly requiring the most training and experience.

- Equilibration alone (unless orthodontics is indicated)
- Orthodontics alone
- Orthodontics and equilibration combination
- Restorative and equilibration combination
- Orthodontic, restorative, and equilibration combination
- Orthognathic surgery, orthodontic, and equilibration combination
- Surgery, orthodontic, restorative, and equilibration combination

REFERENCES

Hannam, A.G., et al. (1977). The relationship between dental occlusion, muscle activity, and associated jaw movement in man. *Archives of Oral Biology*, Vol. 22, pp. 25–32.

Manns, A., Chan, C., and Miralles, R. (1987). Influence of group function and canine guidance on electromyographic activity of elevator muscles. *Journal of Prosthetic Dentistry*, Vol. 57, pp. 494–501.

Manns, A., Miralles, R., and Guerrero, F. (1981). The changes in electrical activity of the postural muscles of the mandible upon varying the vertical dimension. *Journal of Prosthetic Dentistry*, Vol. 45, pp. 438–445.

Manns, A., Miralles, R., and Palazzi, C. (1979). EMG, bite force, and elongation of the masseter muscle under isometric voluntary contractions and variations of vertical dimension. *Journal of Prosthetic Dentistry*, Vol. 42, pp. 674–482.

Riise, C., and Sheikholeslam, A. (1982). The influence of experimental interfering occlusal contacts on the postural activity of the anterior temporal and masseter muscles in young adults. *Journal of Oral Rehabilitation*, Vol. 9, pp. 419–425.

Williamson, E.H., and Lundquist, D.O. (1983). Anterior guidance: Its effect on electromyographic activity of the temporal and masseter muscles. *Journal of Prosthetic Dentistry*, Vol. 49, pp. 816–823.

RECOMMENDED READING

Bakke, M., and Moller, E. (1980). Distortion of maximal elevator activity by unilateral premature tooth contact. *Scandinavian Journal of Dental Research*, Vol. 80, pp. 67–75.

Belser, U.C., and Hannam, A.G. (1985). The influence of altered working-side occlusal guidance on masticatory muscles and related jaw movement. *Journal of Prosthetic Dentistry*, Vol. 53, pp. 406–413.

Crispin, B.J., Myers, G.E., and Clayton, J.A. (1978). Effects of occlusal therapy on pantographic reproducibility of mandibular border movements. *Journal of Prosthetic Dentistry*, Vol. 40, pp. 29–34.

Christensen, L.V., and Rassouli, NM. (1995). Experimental occlusal interferences. Part II. Masseteric EMG responses to an intercuspal interference. *Journal of Oral Rehabilitation*, Vol. 22, pp. 521–531.

Gibbs, C.H., et al. (1984). EMG activity of the superior belly of the lateral pterygoid muscle in relation to other jaw muscles. *Journal Prosthetic Dentistry*, Vol. 51, pp. 691–702.

Hannam, A.G., et al. (1981). The effects of working-side occlusal interferences on muscle activity and associated jaw movements in man. *Archives of Oral Biology*, Vol. 26, pp. 387–392.

Hannam, A.G., and McMillan, A.S. (1994). Internal organization in the human jaw muscles. *Critical Reviews in Oral Biology and Medicine*, Vol. 5, pp. 55–89.

Jimenez, I.D. (1987). Dental stability and maximal masticatory muscle activity. *Journal of Oral Rehabilitation*, Vol. 14, pp. 591–598.

Lund, P., Nishiyama, T., and Moller, E. (1970). Postural activity in the muscles of mastication with the subject upright, inclined, and supine. *Scandinavian Journal of Dental Research*, Vol. 78, pp. 417–424.

Mahan, P.E., et al. (1983). Superior and inferior bellies of the lateral pterygoid muscle EMG activity at basic jaw positions. *Journal Prosthetic Dentistry*, Vol. 50, pp. 710–718.

Radu, M., Marandici, M., and Hottel, T.L. (2004). The effect of clenching on condylar position: A vector analysis model. *Journal of Prosthetic Dentistry*, Vol. 91, pp. 171–179.

Schaerer, P., Stallard, R.E., and Zander, H.A. (1967). Occlusal interferences and mastication: An electromyographic study. *Journal Prosthetic Dentistry*, Vol. 17, pp. 438–449.

Shupe, R.J., et al. (1984). Effects of occlusal guidance on jaw muscle activity. *Journal Prosthetic Dentistry*, Vol. 51, pp. 811–818.

Visser, A., McCarroll, R.S., an Naeije M. (1992). Masticatory muscle activity in different jaw relations during submaximal clenching efforts. *Journal of Dental Research*, Vol. 71, pp. 372–378.

Wood, W.W. (1987). A review of masticatory muscle function. *Journal of Prosthetic Dentistry*, Vol. 57, pp. 222–231.

Evaluating the Muscles of the Stomatognathic System and Their Role in Understanding Occlusal Disharmony and TMD

Herbert E. Blumenthal, DDS

The term *stomatognathic system* as described by Nathan Allen Shore (1976) consists of components of the bones of the upper body from the clavicle upward through the skull; the vascular, lymphatic, and nerve supply systems; the soft tissues of the head; and the teeth. Evaluating a patient's muscles of the stomatognathic system includes observation, history, palpation, and additional diagnostic procedures.

Shore (1976) states, "An organ such as the heart or the liver can be dissected anatomically, but a system such as the stomatognathic must be studied as an integrated, physiological, functioning whole. It is important to consider the specific functions that tie this system together rather than the isolated and individual tissues which compose it."

The stomatognathic system is an integrated complex of parts that are interdependent to the point that dysfunction of one portion can influence the total complex. With a working knowledge of the components of the stomatognathic system, one can evaluate this system as a whole and attempt the most effective examination and correction with minimal effort and trauma to the patient. As dentists, we are primarily concerned with the effects occlusion has on this system. It is our quest to mitigate the

Comprehensive Occlusal Concepts in Clinical Practice, by Irwin M. Becker
© 2011 Blackwell Publishing Ltd.

negative effects that stimulate the adaptive process of the system in an unsuccessful attempt to balance itself.

OCCLUSAL CONNECTION

Establishing wear patterns in the patient's mouth is the best way to determine abnormal muscular involvement. Do you see occlusal evidence of bruxing? When evaluating wear patterns, it is best and most accurate to have correctly mounted study casts with arc of closure registrations along with condylar guidance registration. The steepness of the condylar guidance helps determine the posterior tooth disclusion in lateral and protrusive movements. Prior orthodontic or iatrogenic grinding such as an occlusal equilibration can influence evidence of wear. These factors need to be established before using wear patterns to determine muscle dysfunction.

Of course, the best articulator is the patient. There are limitations in using the patient, especially a patient in pain who will avoid areas of discomfort, giving an inaccurate picture. This can be demonstrated in some patients who have posterior interferences that are mitigated by the use of an anterior deprogrammer. Limited lateral movements without the anterior deprogrammer are very restricted but will immediately free up with the placement of the anterior deprogrammer. Note any muscle trismus when the mandible is moved into a lateral or straight protrusive movement. This is an indicator that there may be interferences within the occlusal scheme that evoke a protective response from the muscles that function to allow this movement to take place.

If one single improper stimulus enters into this complex interdependent system, the entire mechanism is automatically restructured into an adaptive mode in an attempt to accommodate the stimulus. If this is a temporary stimulus, then the system will right itself after the stimulus is removed. The stimulus may be from the periodontal ligament receptors, a neuromuscular spindle cell in a muscle of mastication, iatrogenic tooth position, or muscles of the tongue or hyoid group. A change in the function of the mastication-hyoid complex changes the balancing requirements of the posterior cervical group of muscles.

In an attempt to balance the stomatognathic system, the labyrinthine reflexes can be affected. At times, stimulation of the proprioceptors in the periodontal ligament that fail to return to normal can have far-reaching effects within this system. The chief complaint of the patient may not be the initiating factor in the observable response. This is where our powers of observation and knowledge of how the masticatory system works are invaluable in attempting to determine the cause and effect process.

Note the matching of wear patterns of the mandibular and maxillary teeth. When putting the patient in these positions, note any report of muscular pain. Remember, the patient can put five to nine times more force on the teeth when bruxing as when consciously articulating the teeth together. There may be evidence of excursive interferences, especially after immediately leaving the rotational stage of condyle function. There may be evidence of hypo-occlusion on the same side or hyperocclusion on the opposite side. Involvement of the deep masseter may be due to retrusive inclines and/or retrusive forces in lateral excursion.

Because of the almost limitless combinations of circumstances, the occlusal connections described for each muscle are not by any means limited to what is described in the following text, but I have observed them as possible connections.

THE INITIAL INTERVIEW

The observation process begins during first contact with the patient. Greeting each new patient as she or he is escorted to the conference room offers opportunity to note the patient's standing posture, how the patient interacts with others, the position of the head during standing and walking, shoulder positions, arm-length discrepancy, and other imbalances that are best observed when the patient is not seated. An understanding of the cause and effect of any structural imbalance on occlusal disharmony and TMD (temporomandibular joint disorder) will be developed while taking an in-depth history and conducting a physical examination.

Figure 6.1 illustrates some physical observations that may be made. Note in this image the patient's head position, that she carries her purse on her right shoulder, the unequal height of her shoulders, and how the patient is placing most of her weight on her right leg.

During the initial interview, ask questions about the patient's history. My assistant takes notes so I can focus on watching the patient respond to questions. Questions about complaints often stimulate body movements that provide clues for additional questions. Because patients tend to talk only about what they think is relevant, it is helpful to explain that symptoms sometimes have far-reaching effects and seemingly irrelevant information could be relevant. Ask the patient to share all experienced symptoms.

The recorded history will guide questioning and observation prior to the physical examination. The following symptoms are common to TMD patients and are likely to be mentioned when you question your patient:

- Frequent headaches
- Facial pain
- Pain when chewing
- Pain in jaw joint(s)
- Noises in jaw joint(s) when moving or chewing
- Limited opening of mouth

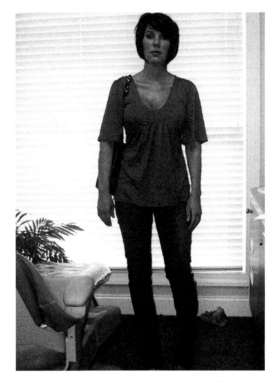

Fig. 6.1. Structural imbalance associated with occlusal disharmony.

- Jaw locks
- Awareness of clenching or grinding of teeth
- Neck pain
- Shoulder pain
- Sensitive teeth
- Ear pain
- Ringing in ear(s)
- Face gets tired when chewing
- Pain behind eyes

If there are multiple complaints, I might ask, "If we could fix one thing and one thing only for you today, what would you choose?" The answer tells me what annoys the patient most. The question may remove the patient's preconceived ideas of what might be important. Even if what the patient would like fixed most surprises me, I make sure to address it in the examination process.

At the end of the initial interview, I ask the patient if there is anything we did not talk about that I should know. I ask the patient if there is anything she or he would like to know about me or about our office.

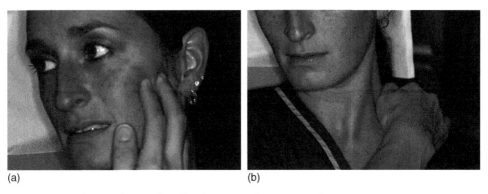

(a)   (b)

Figs. 6.2a and 6.2b. Patient touching areas of pain.

OBSERVATIONS TO MAKE DURING THE INITIAL INTERVIEW

What Areas Does the Patient Touch When Describing the Pain or Chief Complaint? (See figs. 6.2a and 6.2b.)

The patient will touch the area(s) that are most affected. When the patient says he or she has TM joint pain, does the patient specifically point to the joint, or does the patient use a circular motion outlining a muscular component? Many times, the patient is outlining the masseter (superficial and/or deep), posterior digastric, attachment of the sternocleidomastoid to the mastoid process, or the temporalis attachment to the coronoid process. This area may exhibit vascular pain from one of several branches of the carotid artery. Do not draw conclusions, but rather make observations that will be a part of the overall initial diagnosis.

Note pain progression patterns indicated by the movement of the patient's hands. For example, the patient may manually trace pain starting in the neck and moving to the face. This can be extremely helpful in identifying referred pain patterns. Most patients do this automatically while in the process of verbally describing their discomfort, but this often goes unnoticed as a diagnostic tool. Note that the origin of pain may not be the initiating point of the problem.

Does the Patient Mention a Noise or Feeling in the Jaw Joint(s)?

If the patient describes a noise in the jaw joint(s), ask the patient to reproduce the noise, and note what the patient does with his or her mandible to reproduce it. The patient has lived with this for some time and knows exactly what to do to reproduce the dysfunction of the joint(s). Note the position of the mandible in relationship to the maxilla and the position of the head and neck when the patient is demonstrating this position. It may require a series of mandibular movements for the patient to reproduce the noise and feeling. Later, during the clinical examination, look for physical signs that this event takes place. There may be evidence of tooth wear, pain, or tooth mobility to support this position. Be aware that the noise and pain in the joints may not coincide.

What Does the Patient Do with Her or His Teeth while Describing the Chief Complaint?

Observe what the patient is doing with his or her mouth during the initial interview. Is the patient talking with teeth closed together? Look and listen for a tongue thrust producing a lateral or intradental lisp. This is an indicator of myofunctional dysfunction. A patient who keeps teeth together in an inappropriate way does so for a reason. Look for the patient positioning the mandible forward while talking. Look for avoidance patterns. Reasons for positioning the mandible in an awkward position may be avoidance of tooth pain, joint pain, muscle pain, or a combination of these.

What is the relationship of the mandibular and maxillary teeth when noise and/or pain is generated in the joint(s)? What muscles are used to position the mandible to reproduce this noise or pain? The lateral pterygoid muscles are partially responsible for lateral/straight protrusive and opening the mandible. The digastric muscles are additional primary opening and guiding muscles in the lateral protrusive and are often responsible for what the patient describes as ear pain, both direct and referred.

How Does the Patient Position the Head to Reproduce the Pain?

What muscles are being used to reproduce the pain response? What agonist and antagonist muscles are involved? Note the position of the mandible. Are teeth hitting in an inappropriate way in this position? Are these teeth the same ones that have been reported as sensitive or painful? Evaluate the position of the head and neck, and establish how this position may occur.

When you ask the patient to reproduce tooth pain, what does the patient do? Patients who have unusual tooth pain may only be able to reproduce this pain when they go into a parafunctional position. Often tooth mobility can only be explained in response to a parafunctional position. Obtaining this posture requires muscle contraction. If possible, make the connection for the patient by pointing out the relationship of the position to the symptom.

Asking the patient to reproduce muscle discomfort will often also reproduce the tooth problem. Conversely, tooth pain may only be reproduced when the head and neck are in an awkward position. This offers an opportunity to involve the patient in a codiscovery process. Be careful not to come to any conclusions at this point, but only observe and record the information. An in-depth examination will be done following the initial interview to confirm the connection.

Many times patients will seek out awkward positions just to get the teeth to contact that have become sensitive or painful. Awkward head and neck positions involving agonist and antagonist muscles most likely accompany parafunctional positions of the mouth. Sometimes these connections are found during awkward sleeping patterns, unusual working positions or cradling a telephone. How does the patient communicate with you? Is the patient exhibiting awkward head, neck, or facial positions during normal conversation? Do any of these positions involve muscles, exhibiting pain patterns? Use this information to help guide the physical examination to confirm subjective findings.

Figure 6.3 was extracted from a video of an initial interview with the patient. She was answering a question. The information gained from this photograph was invaluable in determining the etiology of specific muscle discomfort she was experiencing in her facial musculature.

In figure 6.4, the patient was asked to clench her teeth as hard as she could. Note the involvement of the neck muscles in the clenching process. Be aware that especially women tend to clench their teeth several times

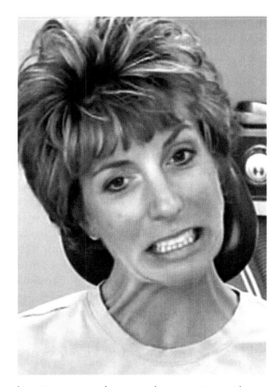

Fig. 6.3. Head position occurred in normal conversation with patient.

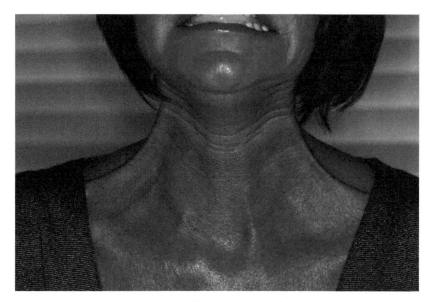

Fig. 6.4. Patient clenching teeth as hard as she could clench.

harder while sleeping than when awake. Note the involvement of the platysma muscle. This muscle involvement is often overlooked in the clenching and bruxing process.

Do You Observe Asymmetry?

It is important to note any asymmetry of the head and neck. I find it helpful to note the symmetry of the nostril openings. A compromised opening usually indicates asymmetrical growth that could be significant in determining muscular patterns.

The patient in figure 6.5 was asked to sit up in a relaxed position. Note the sternocleidomastoid (SCM) muscles, both the sternal and the clavicular portion of the muscles, and how much contraction there is on both sides. Contraction occurs when the patient has a forward head position putting stress on the agonist and antagonist muscles of the SCM. The antagonist muscles for the SCM are the spinalis capitis, splenius capitis, and semispinalis capitis, among others. These muscles, within the parameters of dental protocol, are identifiable during the clinical examination. If the SCM muscles stay in a state of abnormal contraction for an extended time, their effect can cascade throughout the entire system.

Does the Patient Have Any Visible Scars?

Ask about scars on the patient's face and any visible portion of the body. Often a patient will not remember traumas or accidents until you ask. It's

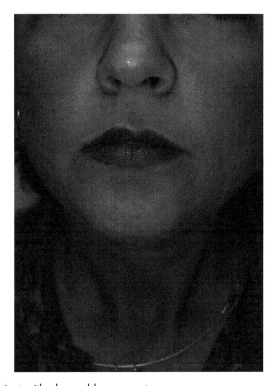

Fig. 6.5. Patient with observable asymmetry.

not uncommon for a patient to call the office after the initial visit to report recalled events. The patient might describe the pain beginning on or about the time they were involved in an accident. Although a connection may be obvious to you, it may not register with the patient. You may need to ask, "Do you think there may be a connection between the accident and the symptoms you are having?" If you involve the patient in the discovery process, the process becomes a joint effort and is much easier.

When turning his or her head to the right or left, does the patient feel restricted? Does the patient use neck muscles or recruit the shoulder and upper back muscles to make the movement? Restricting muscles can be explored and identified later in the examination process. Note the neck muscles when the patient is sitting in a relaxed position. Are the SCM muscles contracting inappropriately? Note the overall musculature of the face.

What Is the Patient's Position while Sleeping and Working?

Some patients who sleep on their stomachs have muscular tension from turning their head to one side, referring pain to the head and neck. Others experience neck and shoulder tension while working at their desk. Where are the patient's arms when using a computer keyboard? What are the heights of the patient's desk and chair? Sleep and work positions can be modified once the patient is aware of their destructive forces.

How Does the Patient Rate Individual Symptoms?

Chronic pain patients usually have multiple factors contributing to their symptoms. As some problems begin to resolve, other problems begin to surface. It is worthwhile to explain this possibility to the patient. I find it helpful to have patients fill out a form at the beginning, which later reminds them of their original complaint and allows them to evaluate their progress. Patients complete this form each time they return for an appointment. The original is sent to the referring professional and a reduced copy is kept in the record.

On this form, each symptom is listed, and the patient evaluates each symptom by indicating whether it is no longer present (NLP), better (B), same (S), or worse (W). The patient is invited to note comments or items for discussion at that visit. Responses are tracked for the entire time a splint is worn. Also included on the sheet is an analog scale that indicates 0 to 10, 0 being where the patient started at the first visit and 10 being perfect. This information becomes part of the patient's permanent record. As the symptoms begin to resolve, the corresponding agonist and antagonist muscles should also respond.

The patient is given a full body drawing to mark where pain occurs. This presents an opportunity for the patient to understand that the problem may extend beyond the teeth and jaw. Many times patients will mark no headaches on the history form, but when questioned directly, they state that they do have headaches that are "normal" headaches not related to their teeth. This is one question that you may want to ask regardless of the answer given on the history form. Many times patients attribute their headaches to sinus problems or "migraine" headaches. When asked directly about the migraine headaches, most times they do not fit the criteria for migraines but are more likely muscular contraction or referred pain pattern type headaches.

What Are the Patient's Expressions During General Conversation?

It is interesting to observe pain responses that are initiated by events described by the patient. An example would be someone who has a severe muscular response causing initiation of the symptoms when describing a physical or emotional trauma. This should be noted and taken under consideration for future reference. Perhaps help from outside the dental profession may be needed. I have learned not to be quick in making final decisions about a diagnosis. Each time the patient returns to the office, there is an opportunity to rediagnose the circumstances.

Is the Patient Dependent on Another Person to Answer Questions?

If the patient is dependent on others during the initial visit, this could be a sign of psychological problems. You may not be gathering all of the information you need and should move slowly on diagnosis. Later, during treatment, this same patient may not respond to treatment as expected and you will again consider the possibility of psychological influences.

Although an inappropriate response to treatment may be a sign of problems that merit psychological consultation, we still must be careful not to categorize all inappropriate responses to treatment as psychological in origin. An unexpected response may mean that we do not clearly understand the scope of involvement of the initiating factors and that we should consider changes in our approach. But the negative response could be episodic and not represent a trend. If we make adjustment to the appliance to accommodate an unexpected response, we must consider if we are adapting the appliance to only an episodic response. For example, a patient has been responding well to splint therapy and returns to your office with a severe headache or other symptoms following an incident. In these cases, it is sometimes best not to adjust the splint to these circumstances. Only if symptoms do not resolve in a reasonable time should one consider the adjustment process. This is a difficult call and should be done only with considerable thought about the overall process.

An unexpected response may be another opportunity to explore the possibility that you may need help from other professionals. Many times we can take the patient only so far with splint therapy. Basically we are tricking the brain into thinking that the patient has an ideal bite relationship and that the protective muscular response is not necessary. Many times physical therapy and other modalities are needed. It works best to coordinate your adjustment appointment immediately following the outside therapy. Have the therapist place cotton rolls between the patient's teeth and keep them there until the patient returns to your office (*assuming the appointments are coordinated to follow one another*). When the patient returns to your office, remove the cotton rolls, have the patient insert the splint, and check the occlusion. Adjustments are most effective when done this way because you are adjusting the bite to a corrected position of the system. This will be discussed in more detail in later chapters of this book.

Is Your Written History Flexible Enough to Include the Unexpected?

Let your patient talk. The patient has lived with the problem for an extended time and has information that can help solve the mystery. Many times I will ask the patient, "If you had the ability to do anything you needed to do, what would you do to fix the problem?" Sometimes I have been surprised by the answer. It is the practitioner's quest to assimilate this information and put it into a usable format to piece together the puzzle. Allow your history taking to be flexible enough to explore unexpected avenues presented by the patient.

THE INITIAL PHYSICAL EXAMINATION OF THE MUSCLES

Using the definition of the stomatognathic system, the entire process of evaluation and initial diagnosis should be expanded to include the musculature listed below. I have chosen muscles that are within the scope of dental protocol for examination and evaluation. These muscles go beyond what we have traditionally learned as the muscles of mastication: temporalis, masseter, digastric, medial, and lateral pterygoid. The expanded examination process considers the agonist and antagonist muscles.

It is important to note that muscles do not turn on or off. They do, however, change their contractual state as is demonstrated by the increase or decrease in electromyographic readings. The agonist muscles are anatomically attached so when they contract they develop forces that reinforce each other. The antagonist muscles generate opposing forces when contracting.

There is a dance among the primary muscles, their agonist and antagonist to produce a smooth and controlled, predictable movement of bones. Repeated interruption of the normal process introduces the probability of dysfunctional movement. For example, muscle trismus upon left or right protrusive movements can be an attempt of the system to protect itself. Dysfunctional movements may be so subtle that they are not detectable by observation. Given enough time, these patterns or results of these patterns may become clinically observable.

Decrease of vertical opening may be due to muscle restriction of the opening or closing muscles. One cannot make the assumption that the primary functional muscle is the one that is causing the restrictive or altered movements. For example, if the masseter muscle is restricting the vertical opening, releasing the digastric and inferior lateral pterygoid muscles may immediately release the masseter, compensating contraction as an antagonist muscle to the opening muscles.

The human being is a closed kinematic chain. Stimulation of one part of the body affects every portion of the body in some way. One must grasp the connection of the agonist-antagonist relationships before reaching conclusions about muscle dysfunction. There are many reasons for muscle dysfunction. Some of these may be beyond the scope of dentistry but must not be ignored.

The infrahyoid and suprahyoid muscles should be part of the expanded examination process. Along with the posterior neck muscles, they provide direct support to the process of mastication and other functional movements of the mandible. One must take into consideration that the movements of the mandible are not usually predictable in an exact pathway.

The mandible has a range of movements. Even though the muscle contraction in primary, agonist, and antagonist cannot easily be specifically patterned, one can expect certain patterns to occur within an intentional range of motion. In the case of a ginglymo-arthrodial joint, the possible combinations of movement are almost limitless. While one side is hinging, the other side may be in a protrusive movement using a different set of muscles.

When the mandibular and maxillary dentition is in contact, there is a great complexity of muscular inhibition and contraction to stabilize the hyoid bone. Even in the movement of the tongue during chewing and swallowing, there is involvement of the suprahyoid and infrahyoid musculature to help maintain hyoid stability.

The following descriptions of muscles take into consideration the primary and secondary function. This does not preclude the possibility that eccentric movements could give an altered picture of combinations of agonist and antagonist muscles.

THE TEMPORALIS MUSCLE

Primary Action: The primary action of the temporalis is traditionally described as the elevation of the mandible when acting bilaterally. Although it is described in the literature as a closing muscle, it is primarily a positioning muscle. Its three segments, anterior, middle, and posterior, work in concert to help position the condyle-mandible assembly in closing, opening, lateral protrusive, and retrusive. This muscle is active throughout the entire range of mandibular movements.

Origin and Insertion: The origin of the temporalis muscle is the temporal fossa and temporal fascia. The insertion of the muscle is the coronoid process and the ramus of the mandible (fig. 6.6).

Primary Action Agonists: There are many muscles that can work as both agonist and antagonist muscles. The digastric muscle, along with the lateral pterygoid muscle, works in this way with the temporalis muscle. The muscles that work as agonist in harmony with the temporalis are the masseter and medial pterygoid. The temporalis muscle acts as a guide for these power-closing muscles. During retrusion of the mandible, the digastric muscle and the superior portion of the lateral pterygoid work in concert with the posterior fibers of the temporalis muscle. Observing the function of these muscles offers opportunity to see how muscles are multifaceted in function and not designated to only one function.

Primary Action Antagonists: The posterior belly of the digastric and both the superior and inferior heads of the lateral pterygoid are antagonists to the temporalis during opening and closing. If parafunctional movement occurs when opening the mandible, then the inferior belly of the lateral pterygoid is primarily involved. If parafunctional movement occurs during the closing cycle, then the upper head of the lateral pterygoid is more likely to be involved. A muscle that is often overlooked but seems to be involved

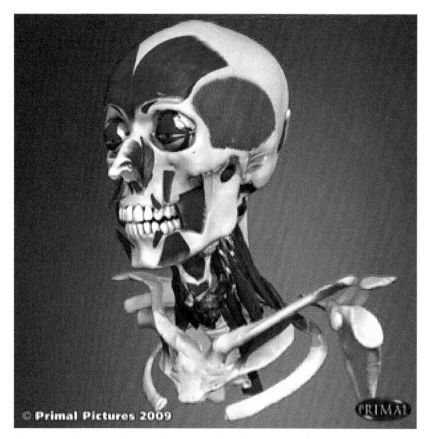

Fig. 6.6. The temporalis muscle. Reprinted with permission from Primal Pictures Ltd (159–165 Great Portland Street; London W1W5PA, UK; www.anatomy.tv).

in multiple functional and parafunctional movements is the platysma muscle.

One cannot isolate specific portions of a muscle to work independently of the rest of the muscle, but certain portions of the muscle may function in a dominant way when attempting to achieve intended positions of the mandible.

When contracted, the anterior portion of the temporalis elevates the condyle apparatus up into the fossa. This can be demonstrated by observing the fibers of the muscle that parallel the fibers of the deep masseter. Both of these muscles are the primary initiators in seating the condyle to stabilize its position in the fossa. This might occur in the rotational stage of arc of closure or if the "system" is attempting to restrict the translation or even the rotational movement of the mandible. When these fibers of the muscle are in parafunction, they may refer pain to upper teeth. This will be discussed later in this chapter.

Secondary Action: The secondary function of the temporalis is retraction of the mandible. This occurs as the posterior aspect of the temporalis contracts bilaterally. Lateral protrusion involves posterior fiber contraction on the side of the lateral movement. The right posterior fibers of the temporalis become active when the mandible is moved to the right to stabilize the condyle in the fossa.

Secondary Action Agonists: The masseter, digastric, medial pterygoid, and superior portion of the lateral pterygoid function as agonist muscles when the temporalis acts bilaterally to retract the mandible. During retraction of the mandible, the temporalis contracts its more horizontal fibers, along with the posterior portion of the digastric. These fibers are located in the posterior portion of the temporalis and the posterior portion of the digastric. The other agonist muscles appear to stabilize the mandibular position more than function as primary power muscles to perform the movement. The digastric action does not initiate in one specific portion of the muscle but ripples from anterior to posterior, ending with the posterior portion of the muscle exhibiting most movement. The picture becomes more complex when one considers the function of the digastric and its relationship to the suprahyoid and infrahyoid muscles. More details of this will be outlined when describing the digastric muscle.

The masseter, contralateral medial pterygoid, contralateral lateral pterygoid, and several of the infrahyoid and suprahyoid muscles act as agonists when the temporalis muscle moves the mandible laterally to right and left protrusive.

Secondary Action Antagonists: The antagonist muscles involved in lateral protrusive movements are the ipsilateral medial pterygoid and ipsilateral lateral pterygoid. The temporalis assists with lateral deviation of the mandible by contracting its anterior fibers only.

Palpation: Before beginning palpation, I explain to patients that it is not necessary to hurt them to find out what I need to know. I demonstrate on a hand or arm the amount of pressure I will use to palpate the muscles. This can be demonstrated by putting enough pressure with your index finger to blanch the fingernail bed, about 3–5 pounds of pressure. When a trigger point of tenderness is found, the patient may think you are putting excessive pressure on that area. If that occurs, I ask the patient to press on that particular area to see how little pressure it takes to evoke a pain response. This is always a learning opportunity for the patient and helps the patient become involved in the examination process.

To begin palpation, place the hand over the ear. The lateral border of the hand is over the external auditory meatus. Spread the fingers upward about one-half inch apart toward the orbital rim. This generally outlines the temporalis muscle. Begin palpating with the index finger at the orbital rim and move posterior following the outline of the middle portion of this muscle as it is attached to the skull. This muscle transitions from the anterior fibers consisting of approximately the first quarter of the entire muscle. The anterior fibers of the muscle are vertical fibers. As you move from the

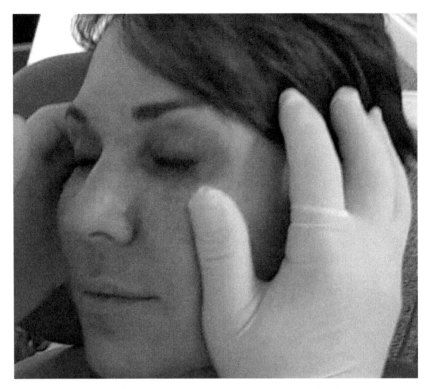

Fig. 6.7. Palpation of temporalis muscle from the anterior index finger at anterior portion.

distal border of the anterior fibers toward the apex of the ear, you are outlining the middle fibers of the temporalis. These fibers are oblique. Continue to move laterally and posterior to the distal extension of the muscle, which is the posterior portion of the temporalis. The posterior fibers are horizontal (fig. 6.7).

Ask the patient to report any muscle tenderness. Areas of tenderness are usually trigger points. These points can be found consistently using the palpation technique. Make notation of each trigger point. Be aware that there can be a direct correlation between point tenderness and certain pain patterns in what seem to be remote areas.

When palpating the anterior portion of the temporalis muscle, be aware of the pterion. The pterion is where the frontal, parietal tip of the greater wing of the sphenoid and the temporal bones come together. It is a very thin area of bone, and when palpating this area, it is almost always tender because of the free nerve endings in the dura and the middle meningeal artery. Consistent pain in this area should alert one to a possible neurological problem, and a neurological examination may be appropriate.

Referred Pain Patterns: There are four referred pain patterns associated with the temporalis, producing temporal headaches and pain in teeth. The

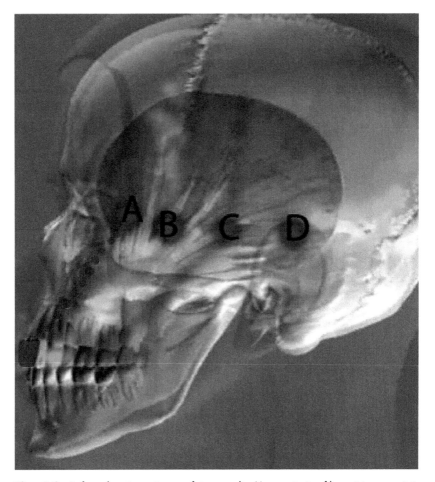

Fig. 6.8. Referred pain patterns of temporalis (A = anterior fibers trigger point, B = middle fibers trigger point, C = posterior fibers trigger point, D = most posterior fibers trigger point).

anterior fibers (A in fig. 6.8) refer pain to the eyebrow and above the trigger point within the temporalis. The middle fibers (B in fig. 6.8) refer pain to the upper premolar area and just above the trigger point. The posterior fibers (C in fig. 6.8) can refer pain to the upper posterior molar teeth. The most posterior trigger point of the temporalis (D in fig. 6.8) will refer pain directly up and slightly posterior to the trigger point.

Innervation: The innervation of the temporalis is the deep temporal branches of the anterior trunk of the mandibular division of the trigeminal nerve.

Blood Supply: The blood supply to the temporalis is the middle temporal branches of the superficial temporal artery and the anterior and posterior deep temporal branch of the maxillary artery.

Possible Occlusal Connection: The anterior portion of the temporalis muscle is possibly affected by excursive interferences in the bicuspid area. The posterior portion of the temporalis muscle (D in fig. 6.8) is most influenced by introduction of retrusive inclines and/or retrusive forces.

THE MASSETER MUSCLE

Primary Action: The primary action of the masseter is the elevation of the mandible. Both the superficial portion (A in fig. 6.9) and deep portion (B in fig. 6.9) of the muscle contracts in this function, but the primary power portion of the muscle is the superficial segment. The deep portion of the masseter contracts along with the anterior fibers of the temporalis and several other muscles to help stabilize the condyle during the movement of the mandible. It also functions in the lateral movement of the mandible

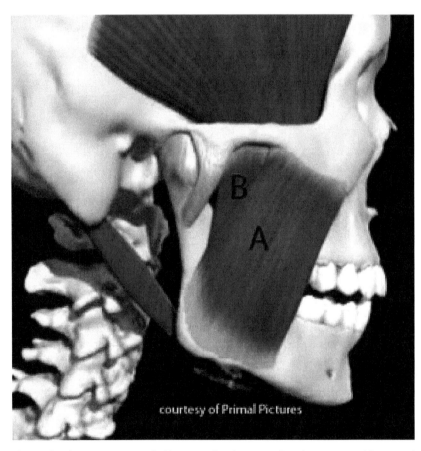

courtesy of Primal Pictures

Fig. 6.9. The masseter muscle (A = superficial portion, B = deep portion.) Reprinted with permission from Primal Pictures.

along with protrusion and retrusion of the mandible. Each of these functions has its own set of agonist and antagonist muscles.

Origin and Insertion: The origin of the superficial portion of the masseter is the anterior and inferior border of the zygomatic arch. This muscle's insertion is the angle and ramus of the mandible. The deep portion origin is distal to the zygomatic suture. The insertion attaches to the coronoid process and the ramus of the mandible. The primary action of the deep portion of the masseter is to seat the condyle along the articular eminence and to help seat the condyle in the fossa. This can be confirmed by the direction of the fibers and the action in an agonist and antagonist function of the muscle.

Primary Action Agonists: The agonist muscles of the deep masseter in the primary action of closure are the anterior fibers of the temporalis and the medial pterygoid. Agonists of the deep layer of the masseter for retrusion of the mandible are the posterior portions of the temporalis. Agonists of the superficial layer of the masseter during mandibular elevation are the contralateral masseter and, bilaterally, the temporalis, medial pterygoid, and superior division of the lateral pterygoid muscles.

Primary Action Antagonists: The antagonist muscles of the deep masseter in the primary action of closure are the digastric and the upper and lower heads of the lateral pterygoid, depending on the position and direction of movement of the condyle. During retrusive, antagonists include the infrahyoid and suprahyoid muscles, including the omohyoid, the anterior belly of the digastric, and the inferior division of the lateral pterygoid. During mandibular elevation, the superficial layer of the masseter has briefly as its antagonist the lower portion of the lateral pterygoid.

Palpation: Palpation of the superficial masseter can be accomplished by dividing the muscle into thirds. With the index and middle finger, palpate from the anterior to the posterior border in each segment. Note that this muscle can have several trigger points with their own specific pain referral patterns. Palpation of the deep masseter can be accomplished by having the patient open wide. Place the index finger over the coronoid notch. Once in this position, press medially (fig. 6.10).

The masseter is an indicator muscle for parafunctional activities, primarily clenching, which may be initiated by an arc of closure interference, and bruxing in lateral or straight protrusive movements of the mandible. Lateral and protrusive bruxing patterns may have a variety of initiators.

Referred Pain Patterns: The masseter may refer pain to the maxilla and above the eyebrow, upper posterior teeth, and lower posterior teeth. The deep portion of the masseter may refer pain directly to the temporomandibular joint and surrounding structures, including the ear, and to the body of the mandible. The referred pain to the teeth may include sensitivity to pressure and temperature changes. Associated trigger points may develop in the ipsilateral temporalis, medial pterygoid, and masseter muscles. These are agonist muscles during the bruxing pattern.

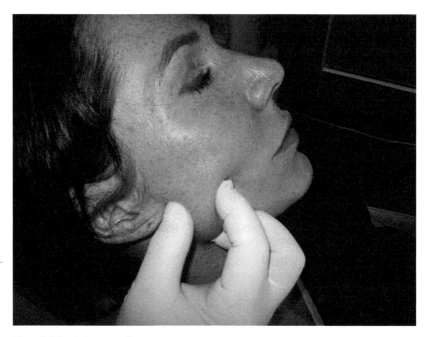

Fig. 6.10. Palpation of masseter.

These patterns may cascade through the stomatognathic system, including the SCM and its associated agonist and antagonist.

Numerous studies have shown that the masseter is one of the most commonly involved muscles in producing trigger points associated with facial pain (fig. 6.11). It has been my observation that the attachment of the temporalis at the coronoid process and the medial pterygoid is also involved in this pain pattern but not reported by the patient. Often, the examination of the ipsilateral lateral pterygoid from within the oral cavity is, in fact, palpation of the attachment of the temporalis at the coronoid process and the medial pterygoid. Tenderness in the attachment of the temporalis is often mistaken for tenderness of the lateral pterygoid.

The masseter muscles are among the first to contract in persons who are in a state of extreme emotional tension or intense determination. It has been my observation that the attachment of the temporalis at the coronoid process and the medial pterygoid is also involved in this pain pattern but not reported by the patient. Often the examination of the ipsilateral lateral pterygoid from within the oral cavity is, in fact, palpation of the attachment of the temporalis at the coronoid process and the medial pterygoid. Tenderness in the attachment of the temporalis is often mistaken for tenderness of the lateral pterygoid.

Innervation: The innervation to the masseter is the masseteric nerve from the anterior trunk of the mandibular division of the trigeminal nerve.

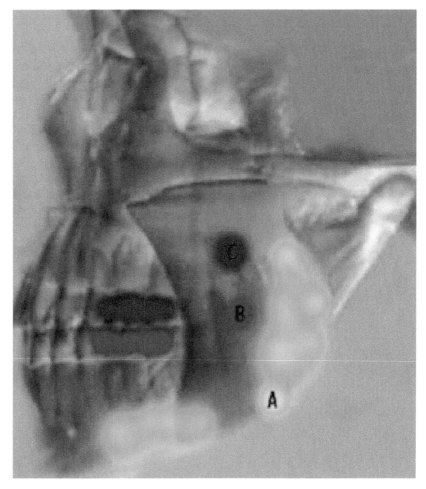

Fig. 6.11. Superficial and deep referred pain patterns of masseter (A = inferior, B = middle, C = superior portion).

Blood Supply: The blood supply to the masseter is the transverse facial branch of the superficial temporal, masseteric branch of the maxillary and the muscular branches of the facial nerve.

Possible Occlusal Connection: The muscular response to these stimuli is accentuated when there is a noxious stimulus. The superficial masseter may be affected by excursive interferences, especially immediately leaving maximum intercuspation of the teeth. If there is unilateral muscular pain, contact of the posterior teeth on the same side as the pain is unlikely. If there is hyperocclusion, then there may be pain on the opposite side. The deep masseter may exhibit excursive interferences due to iatrogenic retrusive contacts or retrusive forces in lateral excursions.

THE LATERAL PTERYGOID MUSCLE

The lateral pterygoid has two divisions, the superior division and the inferior division. Although the two divisions function differently, they are both classified as lateral pterygoid divisions (fig. 6.12).

Action: The lateral pterygoid functions, along with other muscles, as an opening muscle during the opening cycle of the mandible and as a closing and agonist muscle during the closing cycle of the mandible. The lateral pterygoid may function as a supporting muscle to hold the condyle against the incline of the eminence during mouth closure.

Origin and Insertion: The superior portion of the lateral pterygoid arises from the orbital lip of the greater wing of the sphenoid bone. The inferior portion of the lateral pterygoid arises from the lateral surface of the lateral pterygoid plate.

The fibers of the superior portion of the lateral pterygoid insert on the articular disk of the temporomandibular joint and into the upper part of the pterygoid fovea, forming a portion of the superior joint space of the temporomandibular joint (fig. 6.13). Approximately 15% of the fibers attach to the articular disc, and 85% attach to the upper portion of the pterygoid fovea. Results of EMG studies indicate that, in most subjects, the inferior head contracts on opening, and the superior head is electrically active during closing.

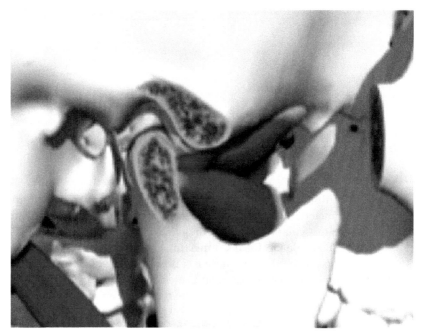

Fig. 6.12. The lateral pterygoid muscle. Reprinted with permission from Primal Pictures.

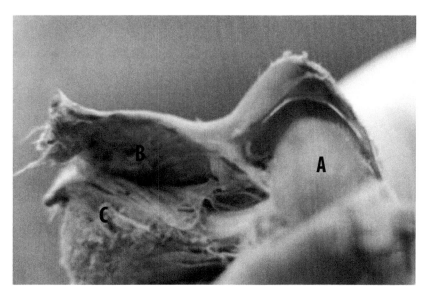

Fig. 6.13. The lateral pterygoid muscle (A = condylar head, B = superior lateral pterygoid, C = inferior lateral pterygoid).

The fibers of the inferior portion of the lateral pterygoid insert into the pterygoid fovea of the mandible (fig. 6.13).

Agonists: The agonist muscles of the lateral pterygoid change with movement of the mandible. Straight vertical opening of the mandible is a bilateral function of the inferior belly of the lateral pterygoid, working in cooperation primarily with the digastric, medial pterygoid, and platysma. The infrahyoid muscles help to stabilize the hyoid bone and act as a force to allow the digastric to apply vector forces necessary to open vertically.

Electromyographic evidence shows the activity of the inferior belly of the lateral pterygoid is decreased when the condyle is in the rotational stage and increased during the opening or translation stage of opening.

When moving in a straight protrusive movement, the inferior belly of the lateral pterygoid works as the primary agonist along with the masseter and temporalis. In lateral protrusive movements, the inferior belly of the lateral pterygoid functions in cooperation with the contralateral digastric (primarily anterior portion of the muscle), medial pterygoid (both ipsilateral and contralateral), masseter (both ipsilateral and contralateral), and temporalis (both ipsilateral and contralateral).

Antagonists: In both vertical opening and protrusive, the inferior and superior bellies of the lateral pterygoid also function as antagonists, depending on the movement of the mandible. When the mandible begins to return to its neutral position in the glenoid fossa, the superior belly of the lateral pterygoid coordinates and takes over the primary action of the muscular to increase in electromyographic readings as the inferior belly decreases in readings.

Palpation: Palpation of the superior and inferior lateral pterygoid muscles has generated some controversy. Some say, and I agree, that these muscles cannot be palpated directly. It has been my experience after three dissection classes that one cannot directly palpate these muscles. At best, one is palpating the space that these muscles function within and most likely palpating the coronoid process at the attachment of the temporalis muscle and the medial pterygoid muscle. If the inferior belly of the lateral pterygoid(s) is in spasm, then the lateral pterygoid(s) will evoke a response to the patient being asked to protrude against the pressure placed on the mandible. This can be accomplished by placing your thumb on the symphysis of the mandible to resist the prostrusive movement (fig. 6.14).

Referred Pain Pattern: The superior and inferior lateral pterygoid muscles refer pain to the temporomandibular joint and to the maxillary sinus areas. The inferior belly (A in fig. 6.15) refers pain toward the joint and external auditory meatus. The superior belly of lateral pterygoid muscles (B in fig. 6.15) refers pain toward the orbit.

Innervation: The innervation of the lateral pterygoid muscle is the external pterygoid nerve.

Blood Supply: The blood supply is the pterygoid branch of the maxillary artery.

Possible Occlusal Connection: The lateral pterygoid is involved in almost every movement of the mandible; therefore, it is a candidate for abnormal responses in a variety of circumstances. Please note that this muscle does not work alone, so there will be other muscles involved in any attempt to mitigate an inability to balance the system. The combination of

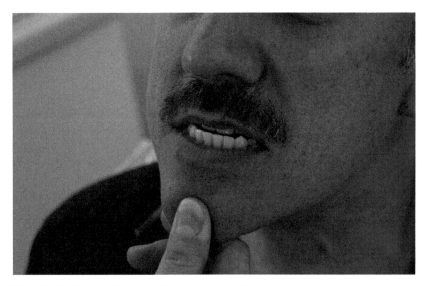

Fig. 6.14. Provocation test of lateral pterygoids.

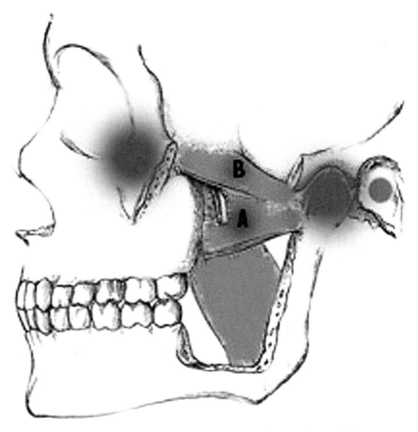

Fig. 6.15. Referred pain patterns of lateral pterygoids (A = inferior belly, B = superior belly).

these muscles will help to identify the possible occlusal connection to the muscular and pain referral pattern.

THE MEDIAL PTERYGOID MUSCLE

Action: This muscle (fig. 6.16) functions to protract and elevate the mandible. It assists in suspending the mandible within the sling formed by itself and the masseter. It also assists in protrusion of the mandible as well as lateral deviation.

Origin and Insertion: The medial pterygoid is attached to the angle of the mandible and to the lateral pterygoid plate. Its origin is the lateral pterygoid plate and its insertion the angle of the mandible.

Agonists: During closing of the mandible, the agonist muscles of the medial pterygoid are the bilateral masseter and temporalis. During

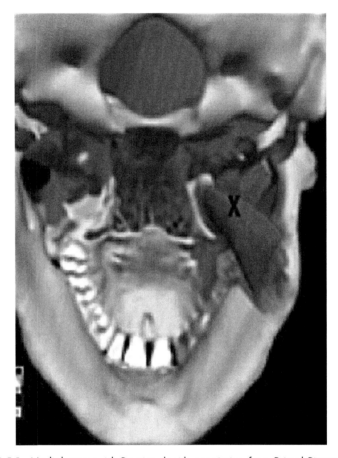

Fig. 6.16. Medial pterygoid. Reprinted with permission from Primal Pictures.

protrusion, when the medial pterygoid is acting bilaterally, the agonist muscles are the upper and lower heads of the lateral pterygoids. When there is contralateral movement of the mandible, the upper and lower heads of the lateral pterygoid act as agonists.

Antagonists: During closing of the mandible, the antagonist muscles of the medial pterygoid are the digastric, upper, and lower heads of the lateral pterygoid and the platysma. During protrusion, when the medial pterygoid is acting bilaterally, the antagonist muscles are the temporalis and digastric. When there is contralateral movement of the mandible, the contralateral muscles act as antagonists.

Palpation: Palpation of the medial pterygoid (fig. 6.17) can be done extraorally by placing the fingers along the inner surface of the mandible at its angle. Intraorally it can be found posterior to the lower molars behind the coronoid process upward toward the medial pterygoid plate. The attachment of the medial pterygoid is along the medial surface of the

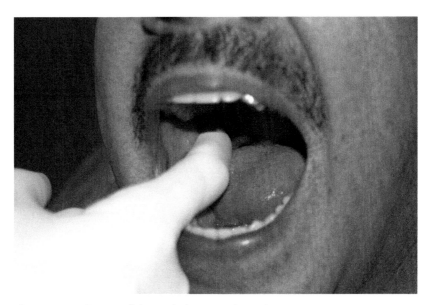

Fig. 6.17. Palpation of the medial pterygoid muscle.

mandible above the angle and to the medial pterygoid plate of the sphenoid bone.

Referred Pain Patterns: The referred pain patterns from the medial pterygoid vary somewhat but usually occur deep in the ear and behind the temporomandibular joint (fig. 6.18). The patient usually will complain of moderate restriction when opening the mandible and may complain about pain when swallowing. Because of its close proximity to the tensor veli palatini, the patient may experience a feeling of stuffiness in the ear if the medial pterygoid impairs the function of the tensor veli palatini to clear the eustachian tube.

Innervation: Innervation of the internal pterygoid is the internal pterygoid nerve from the mandibular division of the trigeminal nerve.

Blood Supply: The blood supply is the muscular branch of the facial pterygoid branches of the maxillary artery.

Possible Occlusal Connection: The occlusal imbalance that affects the medial pterygoid may be most affected by bruxing patterns that involve working and balancing interferences. The imbalance primarily affects the muscle on the same side as the interferences, although both muscles are involved. As a result, one side is more tender. Usually both medial pterygoid muscles are affected by arc of closure interferences. It is difficult to predict which muscles will be most affected by specific interferences since the system attempts to work in the most efficient way it can to avoid problems and may cause unusual movements that are unique to a particular individual.

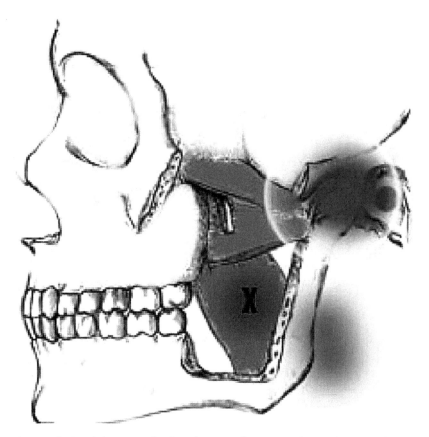

Fig. 6.18. Medial pterygoid referred pain to the joint and ear, also secondary to the posterior border of the mandible.

THE STERNOCLEIDOMASTOID MUSCLE

Action: The clavicular (A in fig. 6.19) and sternal (B in fig. 6.19) portions of the SCM have functions that are cooperative but different. The sternal portion is the closest to the surface. The sternal portion, when acting unilaterally, assists in turning the head. When acting bilaterally, it flexes the head in a forward position. The clavicular portion is the deeper of the two divisions and acts to turn and rotate the skull in an upward position.

Origin and Insertion: The origin of the sternal head attaches to the anterior surface of the sternum. The origin of the clavicular portion attaches to the surface of the medial aspect of the clavicle. The insertion of the SCM muscle is the lateral surface of the mastoid process and the lateral half of the superior nuchal line of the occipital bone.

Agonist and Antagonist: When there is flexion of the head and cervical spine, the agonist is the longus capitis, and the antagonists are the longissimus capitis, spinalis capitis, and the posterior fibers of the SCM.

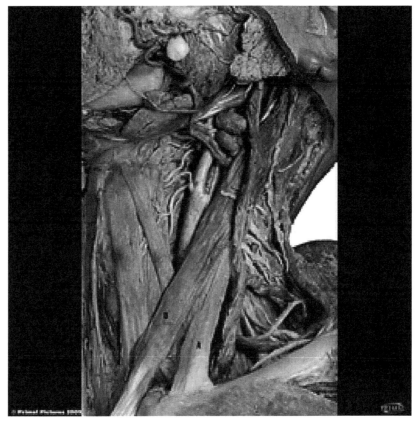

Fig. 6.19. The sternocleidomastoid muscle (SCM; A = clavicular portion, B = sternal portion). Reprinted with permission from Primal Pictures.

When there is lateral flexion of the head, the primary agonist muscle is the splenius capitis, and the antagonist muscles are the same muscles on the opposite side.

During contralateral rotation of the head and cervical spine, when acting unilaterally, the agonist muscle is primarily the semispinalis capitis. The antagonist muscles for this movement are the same muscles on the opposite side: spinalis capitis and trapezius (upper part).

Palpation: If you are standing in front of the patient, grab the SCM muscle, beginning at the insertion at the mastoid process, between the index finger and your thumb (fig. 6.20). Work your way down the muscle toward the clavicular and sternal portion of the muscle. Have the patient report any change in the way one side feels relative to the other side. Note the location of this difference since it can be important in the identification of referred pain patterns.

Referred Pain Patterns: Trigger points along the clavicular portion of this muscle may refer pain to the ear and the frontalis area of the forehead.

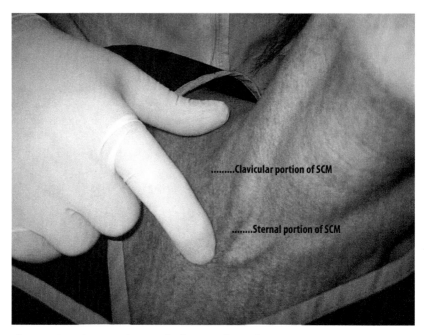

Fig. 6.20. Palpation of sternocleidomastoid muscle.

This pattern is the only one described by Janet Travell (1983) that will cross the midline. The patient will actually touch the place it begins on the frontalis area and trace it across the midline when describing the pain. The patient will say, "It starts here and moves to here." Many times, patients who have looked for treatment for ear pain actually are having referred pain from the clavicular portion of the SCM muscle (fig. 6.21).

The sternal portion of this muscle has a different pain referral pattern. It may be described as pain above the eye and the patient will draw out the pattern when describing pain in the occiput area on the same side as the affected muscle. This portion of the SCM may also refer pain to the upper portion of the sternum at its attachment to the sternum.

Innervation: The innervation of the SCM is the second cervical and spinal portion of the accessory nerve.

Blood Supply: The blood supply is from the SCM branch of the superior thyroid, the occipital branch of the posterior auricular artery, the SCM branch of the occipital artery, and the SCM branch of the suprascapular artery.

Additional Comments: The literature reports that greater than 80% of forward head position patients have a Class II jaw relationship. Forward head position can cause alterations in the stomatognathic system, including change in the muscle activity of the masticatory muscles and dental occlusion. The ramifications of this position can contribute to the manifestation of clinical symptoms such as posterior neck pain, referred pain

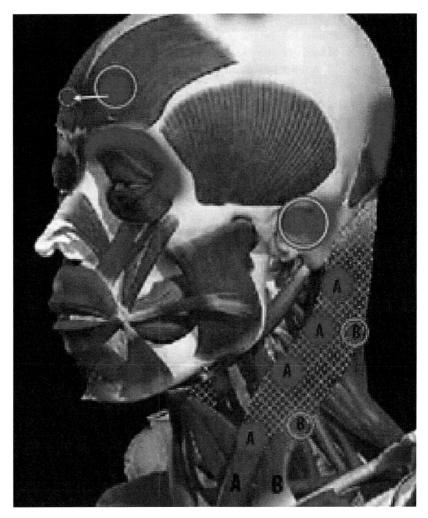

Fig. 6.21. Combined pain patterns of the sternal and clavicular portion of the SCM muscle (A = sternal portion, B = clavicular portion of the SCM, and the clavicular portion has a circle around the referred pain patterns). Reprinted with permission from Primal Pictures.

patterns due to involvement of the suprahyoid and infrahyoid muscles, and also the SCM muscles. Reported symptoms may be the result of referred pain from a secondary location that seems unrelated to the actual etiology.

Carter et al. (1977) and also Cohen (1959) showed through experiments with monkeys that the labyrinth system is oriented to the head in space, while the neck proprioceptors are oriented to the head on the body mechanism. Good (1957) states that the SCM and the upper trapezius muscle can be involved in symptoms of dizziness.

Travell (1983) describes the masseter muscle as having a "satellite" relationship with the SCM muscle. When someone clenches her or his teeth with intensity, the SCM muscle is activated as a stabilizing muscle for the head and neck. This becomes obvious if you ask someone to clench their teeth as hard as they can and watch the SCM muscle along with platysma muscle involvement.

THE DIGASTRIC MUSCLE

The digastric muscle is often overlooked in the TMD examination. This is one of the most used muscles in the function of the mandible. The digastric muscle is best described when comparing it to the reins on a horse. If you want the horse to turn to the right, you tighten the right reins and release the left one. If you want to pull back on the head, you pull back on the reins on both sides.

The digastric muscle is positioned perfectly to act as an opening muscle. Both the anterior portion (A in fig. 6.22) and posterior portion (B in fig.

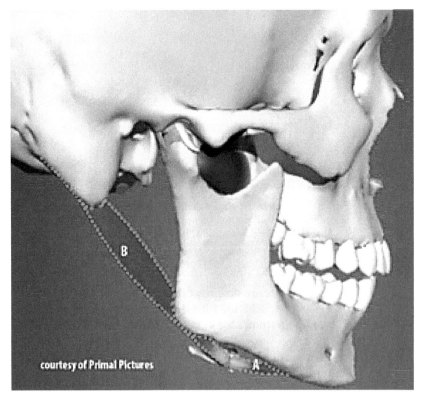

Fig. 6.22. The digastric muscle (A = anterior digastrics, B = posterior digastric). Reprinted with permission from Primal Pictures.

6.22) act in an agonist way to accomplish this movement of the mandible. By contracting bilaterally, the mandible will open vertically. By contracting unilaterally, the mandible will move toward the side of the primary contracting muscle and the opposite digastric acts as an antagonist muscle contraction to regulate the movement of the mandible. It is interesting that the digastric muscle can act as an agonist or antagonist muscle, depending on the function intended.

The digastric muscle also works in harmony with the lateral pterygoid muscles in both an agonist and antagonist fashion. When the digastric muscle contracts bilaterally to open the mandible, the inferior bellies of the lateral pterygoid muscles also contract in an agonist way. The superior belly of the lateral pterygoid muscle acts as an antagonist muscle when the closure muscles begin to take over the function to reverse the opening.

THE DANCE OF THE DIGASTRIC MUSCLE

Beaudreau's group (1969) demonstrated that stimulation of the periodontal ligament receptors, by tapping or chewing, activated the muscles of the hyoid group. This indicates that the digastrics, along with other supra- and infrahyoid muscles, provide a protective mechanism to relieve stress on the dentition during chewing. If there exists noxious stimuli created by malocclusion, it would stand to reason that the supra- and infrahyoid musculature would constantly be activated.

The digastric muscle has a relationship with the inferior lateral pterygoid, superior lateral pterygoid, and the omohyoid muscle in the process of vertical opening and closing as well as lateral and straight protrusive movements. The relationship of these muscles also exists in the reversal of movement of the mandible. The agonist/antagonist muscles work in harmony when reversing the primary intended action, creating a dance among the muscles. When the digastric muscle is involved with the elevation of the hyoid bone, the only way this muscle can function as it does is to be attached to a free-floating bone that allows a great range of motion for the mandible. To stabilize the retraction of the anterior portion of the digastric muscle, the stylohyoid muscle must also be grossly involved in the stabilization of the hyoid to give traction to the contracting muscle to allow movement.

Electromyography appears to clarify the question of which muscles act in mandibular depression. Moyers (1950) found that the lateral pterygoid muscle acts first on jaw opening but is quickly followed by contraction of the anterior belly of the digastric muscle. He concludes that the lateral pterygoid muscle is more responsible for the initiation of the mandibular depression, and the digastric plays an important role in completing the movement.

The right and left digastric muscles always function together, as observed on electromyography. Although the muscles function together bilaterally, the anterior and posterior bellies have independent activities. Munro and Basmajian (1971) found that when the periodontal ligament was stimulated during mastication, the posterior belly of the digastric contracted and the anterior portion of the digastric remained without increased activity. The suprahyoid musculature appears to be important in stabilizing the mandible during all movements.

Munro and Basmajian (1971) summarize the work of several investigators concerning the activity of the digastric muscles in their general function, such as coughing, breathing, chewing, and swallowing. All of these activities strongly recruit the activity of the digastric muscles.

Primary Action: The primary action of the digastric muscle, when acting bilaterally, is depression of the mandible. In the process of depression, the digastric also raises the hyoid bone. This becomes significant when the agonist and antagonist muscles come into play to stabilize the hyoid bone and lend support to the function of the digastric.

Secondary Action: When acting unilaterally, the digastric muscle will reinforce the contralateral lateral pterygoid muscle in assisting the lateral protrusive movement of the mandible to the ipsilateral side of the contraction of the digastric muscle. Another secondary movement is the bilateral contraction to assist the retrusion of the mandible. The movement of the digastric muscle moves the hyoid bone.

Origin and Insertion: The anterior belly of the digastric attaches to the digastric fossa on the inferior border of the mandible. The posterior belly of the digastric attaches to the digastric notch, located in the temporal bone.

Agonists: The agonist muscles for the depression of the mandible are the upper and lower heads of the lateral pterygoid, depending on the direction of the movement of the condylar head within the glenoid fossa. Forward movement activates the lower head of the lateral pterygoid muscle. Backward movement of the condylar head toward the external auditory meatus activates the superior portion of the lateral pterygoid muscle. Movement of the superior and inferior portions must be considered an exchange of activities. Each segment of the lateral pterygoid muscle maintains an electromyographic activity in coordination with its counterpart. As the inferior belly increases in electromyographic activity, the superior belly decreases. As the superior belly increases, the inferior belly decreases in electromyographic activity.

The agonist muscles in the elevation of the hyoid bone are the mylohyoid, geniohyoid, and stylohyoid muscles.

Antagonists: The antagonist muscles involved in the depression of the mandible are medial pterygoid, temporalis, and masseter muscles. The retraction of the mandible involves the following antagonist muscles: lateral pterygoid (mostly the superior head) and the medial pterygoid. When elevating the hyoid bone, the following muscles act as antagonist: omohyoid, sternohyoid, and thyrohyoid.

Palpation: The location of the posterior belly of the digastric in palpation (fig. 6.23) is along a line from the lower anterior aspect of the mastoid

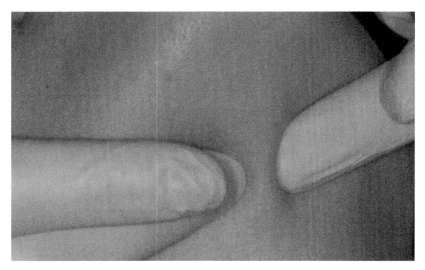

Fig. 6.23. Palpation of the anterior digastric.

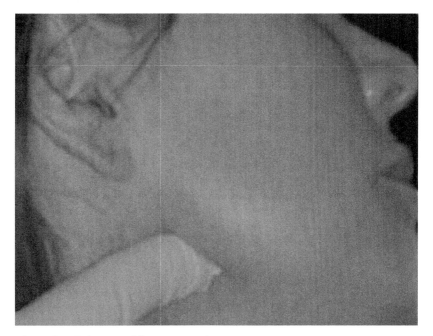

Fig. 6.24. Palpation of the posterior digastric.

process to the upper border of the body of the hyoid. The anterior belly is relatively accessible from the inferior aspect of the mandible (fig. 6.24). The muscle narrows as it approaches the hyoid and goes somewhat laterally.

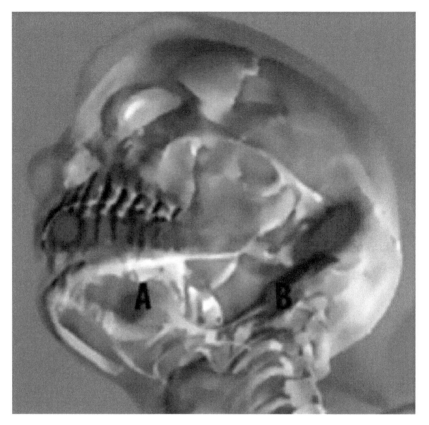

Fig. 6.25. Referred pain patterns of the digastric (A = anterior belly, B = posterior belly). Reprinted with permission from Primal Pictures.

Referred Pain Patterns: The anterior and posterior portions of the digastric have their own referred pain patterns. The posterior portion (B in fig. 6.25) may radiate pain to the upper portion of the SCM muscle, which may radiate to the chin and to the throat. The significance of the referred pain patterns of the anterior portion (A in fig. 6.25) of the digastric muscle is that they may refer pain to the four lower incisors. Awareness of this particular referred pain pattern can often solve a mystery of lower anterior tooth pain that seems to have no apparent dental etiology.

Innervation: The innervation of the digastric muscle is from the digastric branch of the facial nerve.

Blood Supply: The blood supply to the anterior digastric is from the branch of the submental artery off of the external carotid artery. The blood supply to the posterior digastric is from muscular branches of the occipital artery that branch off of the external carotid artery.

Possible Occlusal Connection: The digastric muscle commonly responds when there is a retrusive incline, usually on the anterior teeth, as the digastric becomes overused in an attempt to retract the mandible away from the contact. This is by no means the only circumstance that causes overuse of the digastric muscle, as the digastric muscle is activated each time the mandible deviates to avoid an interference.

THE POSTERIOR NECK MUSCLES

Permission from the patient to examine these muscles should be sought prior to beginning examination. It is not necessary to palpate below the top ridge of the trapezius muscle. The posterior neck muscles are often overlooked in the examination process and can be of great help in recognizing responses to occlusal dysfunction. I have mentioned several times that we are a closed kinematic chain. What affects one part of the body in some way affects the entire system. Most of the time we can and do adapt to these responses and they are of little interest, but it is beneficial to building communication and trust with the patient to codiscover and identify them as much as possible.

Several muscles compose the posterior neck complex, but due to space constraints, only the muscles most accessible for evaluation are described here, beginning with the outermost muscle and working inward toward the spine. These muscles are the trapezius, splenius capitis and cervicis, levator scapula, semispinalis capitis and cervicis, and spinalis capitis and cervicis. Other muscles of interest are the omohyoid, scalene (anterior, middle, and posterior), and several others that can be found described in Gray's Anatomy (1959) and Travell (1983).

THE UPPER TRAPEZIUS MUSCLE

Three segments of the trapezius muscle are described in the literature: upper, middle, and lower portion. The upper portion is described here.

Primary Action: The primary action of the upper trapezius muscle is the rotation of the scapula upward. It also moves the head toward the same side that is contracting and helps to turn the face in the opposite direction. When contracting bilaterally, it draws the head backward (fig. 6.26).

Origin and Insertion: The origin of the upper trapezius muscle is the external occipital protuberance, medial third of the superior nuchal line, the ligmentumm nuchae, and the transverse process of C7. The insertion of the upper trapezius muscle is the lateral third of the clavicle and the medial aspect of the acromion process of the scapula (fig. 6.26).

Agonists: The serratus anterior and the lower part of the trapezius muscle are agonists for the upper trapezius muscle. When the upper trapezius acts to assist the cervical spine extension when acting bilaterally, the agonist muscles involve more of the muscles that would have a direct affect on the stomatognathic system. These muscles are SCM, rectus capitis,

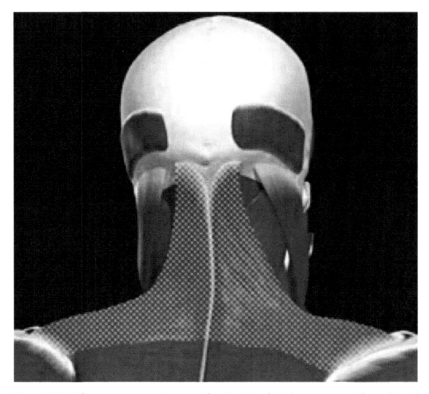

Fig. 6.26. The upper trapezius muscle. Reprinted with permission from Primal Pictures.

splenius cervicis and capitis, longissimus cervicis and capitis, spinalis cervicis and capitis, and semispinalis cervicis and capitis. When assisting with contralateral rotation of the cervical spine and head when acting unilaterally, the agonist muscles are the semispinalis capitis and the SCM.

Antagonists: The antagonist muscles for the upper trapezius muscle are the levator scapulae, serratus anterior, rhomboideus major and minor, and pectoralis major and minor. The antagonist muscles involved in the extension of the cervical spine are longus colli, longus capitis, anterior scalene, and SCM. When the upper trapezius assists in lateral flexion of the cervical spine and acting unilaterally, the agonist muscles are longus colli, rectus capitis, anterior scalene, SCM, splenius cervicis and capitis, and longissimus capitis. The antagonist muscles in this movement are the same muscles on the opposite side.

Palpation: Find the anterior and posterior margins of the upper trapezius muscle at the base of the neck. Grasp the muscle between the index finger and thumb and squeeze. Ask the patient to report any difference in the feeling upon compression. When going through the palpation of any sets of muscles I explain to the patient that I do not have to hurt them to find out what I want to know. To make the process easier to document, I use an analog scale of 0 to 10, 10 being the worst pain they ever had. I let the patient give a number for any feelings they may have upon compression of the muscle. Most discomfort will emerge when compressing any existing trigger points. If the patient gives a number, then it is easier to compare a later reexamination of the same muscle. It is easy to give a percentage difference using the analog scale.

Referred Pain Patterns: Several sources describe the same basic referral pain patterns. Travell (1983) describes the patterns traveling upward from the trigger point to the back of the ear and also to the temporal area behind the eye. The upper trapezius may also refer pain to the occiput area when the trigger point is located more laterally (fig. 6.27).

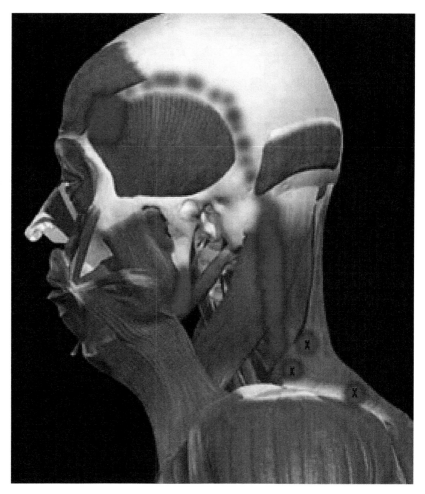

Fig. 6.27. Referred pain patterns of the upper trapezius muscle. Reprinted with permission from Primal Pictures.

Possible Occlusal Connection: The trapezius muscle may be affected by centric relation interferences, especially retrusive inclines. It can also be affected by lack from hypo-occlusion on the ipsilateral side. Postural problems such as forward head position may affect the arc of closure into centric relation by positioning the mandible forward.

THE SPLENIUS CAPITIS MUSCLE

Primary Action: The primary action of the splenius capitis (fig. 6.28), when bilaterally contracting, is to extend the head, laterally flex the head and

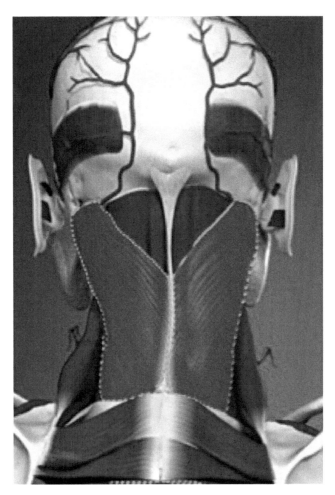

Fig. 6.28. The splenius capitis muscle. Reprinted with permission from Primal Pictures.

neck, and rotate the head slightly when unilaterally contracting. This muscle also acts as a stabilizing muscle for the head and neck. It acts to help counterbalance the forward head position.

Origin and Insertion: The origin of the splenius capitis begins at the lower half of the ligmentum nuchae and the spine of the seventh cervical vertebrae downward to the third or fourth thoracic vertebrae. The insertion of the splenius capitis is into the mastoid process of the temporal bone and travels laterally to part of the superior nuchal line.

Primary Action Agonists and Antagonists: The primary action agonist muscles of the splenius capitis are the longissimus capitis, spinalis capitis, semispinalis capitis, and SCM (posterior fibers). The antagonist muscles of the primary action are the longus capitis and SCM (anterior fibers).

Secondary Action: The secondary action of the splenius capitis is the lateral flexion of the head and cervical spine. The splenius capitis is the only ipsilateral rotator of both the head and cervical spine and does not function in isolation but in conjunction with other rotator muscles.

Secondary Action Agonists and Antagonists: The secondary action agonist muscle is the SCM. The antagonist muscles are the semispinalis capitis and longissimus capitis.

Palpation: Palpating the splenius capitis muscle (fig. 6.29) can be done by locating the depression just below the mastoid process. This identifies the anterior border of the muscle. Move your finger toward the midline

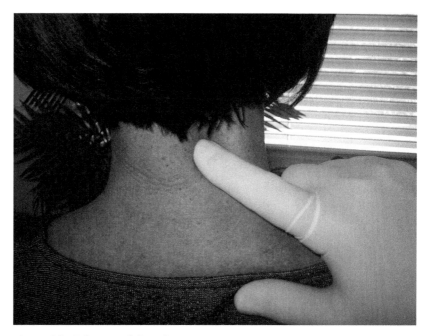

Fig. 6.29. Palpation of the splenius capitis.

from this point to palpate the body of the muscle. If you are not sure if you are on the muscle then have the patient turn their head to the same side you are attempting to palpate the muscle. You should feel the muscle contract with rotation of the skull to the same side as the muscle.

Referred Pain Patterns: The splenius capitis refers pain to the vertex. The splenius capitis can refer pain to the eye and temple area on the same side of the trigger point (fig. 6.30).

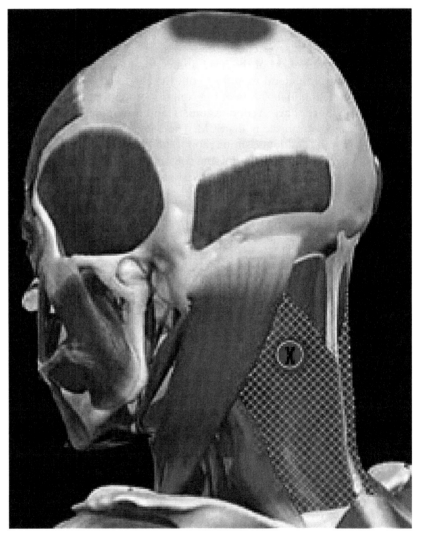

Fig. 6.30. Splenius capitis refers pain to the vertex. Reprinted with permission from Primal Pictures.

Possible Occlusion Connection: The splenius capitis and cervicis may be affected by centric relation arc of closure interferences, especially retrusive inclines.

OTHER FACTORS THAT INFLUENCE MUSCLE FUNCTION

One should not forget the influence of factors other than dental dysfunction that may have a direct or indirect action on the function of the muscles of the stomatognathic system. These may include the following:

- Nutritional factors should be taken into consideration: proper diet, exercise, and most important, proper hydration for the system to function appropriately.
- Medications may block or inhibit the ability to absorb the vitamins, minerals, and amino acids needed to repair and allow muscles to function properly. Medications may alter muscle function as a side effect.
- Sleep disorders are often overlooked as a contributing factor to the overall function and health of the stomatognathic system.
- Psychological factors are very important to consider. Stress can be a major factor in the body's ability to adapt to dysfunction.
- Iatrogenic and congenital changes
- Orthodontics
- Equilibration
- Restorative procedures
- Extractions
- Oral intubation
- Whiplash and other physical injuries
- Growth disturbances
- Arthritis

THE DENTAL ASSISTANT CAN PLAY AN IMPORTANT ROLE

It is essential to have the support of your staff in the overall treatment of TMD patients. My assistant, Pam, has been with me for many years. We work well together, and she knows that she may ask questions anytime she thinks it is appropriate. She was a TMD patient before starting to work with me, so she can answer questions posed by the patient that only someone who has been a TMD patient can appreciate. She is good at explaining procedures to the patient, and because she has been a patient and wears a splint, she can answer most logistical questions. Having someone who is familiar with the wearing of a splint or who has been treated for TMD is a valuable asset. I would suggest that you invite your assistant to undergo a complete examination for TMD and make her or him a splint to wear and experience.

AUTHOR'S COMMENT ON USE OF AN ANTERIOR DEPROGRAMMER

When I was asked to contribute to this book, I was asked to connect tooth wear with muscle function. I realize that that is an impossible task since there are so many factors that are involved. However, one can, in retrospect do just that. One can match tooth wear patterns under pressure and identify which muscles are involved. The patient can do this, and it is a very powerful tool in the codiscovery process. When the only factor initiating the muscular response is an occlusal discrepancy, it can easily be mitigated with the use of an anterior deprogrammer or any device that mitigates the noxious stimulus that has been creating a protective muscular response.

REFERENCES

Beaudreau, D.E., Daugherty, W.F., and Masland, W.S. (1969). Two types of motor pulses in masticatory muscles. *American Journal of Physiology*, Vol. 216.

Carter, B.L., Morehead, J., Wolpert, S.M., et al. (1977). *Cross Sectional Anatomy.* New York: Appleton-Century-Crofts, sections 9–12.

Cohen, L.A. (1959). Body orientation and motor coordination in animals with impaired neck sensation. *Fed Proc*, Vol. 18.

Good, M.G. (1957). Senile vertigo caused by curable cervical myopathy. *Journal of American Geriatric Society*, Vol. 5, pp. 662–667.

Gray, H. (1959). *Anatomy of the Human Body*, 27th ed. Edited by C.M. Goss. Philadelphia: Lea & Febiger.

Moyers, R.E. (1950). An electromyographic analysis of certain muscles involved in temporomandibular movement. *American Journal of Orthodontics*, Vol. 36.

Munro, R.R., and Basmajian, J.V. (1971). The jaw opening reflex in man. *Electromyography*, Vol. 11.

Shore, N.A. (1976). *Temporomandibular Joint Dysfunction and Occlusal Equilibration*, 2nd ed. Philadelphia: J.B. Lippincott.

Travell, J. (1983). *Myofacial Pain and Dysfunction: The Trigger Point Manual.* Baltimore: Williams & Williams.

RECOMMENDED READING

Bjork, A., and Skieller, V. (1972). Facial development and tooth eruption. *American Journal of Orthodontics*, Vol. 62, pp. 339–383.

Bjork, A., and Skieller, V. (1983). Normal and abnormal growth of the mandible: A synthesis of longitudinal cephalometric implant studies over a period of 25 years. *European Journal of Orthodontics*, Vol. 5, pp. 1–46.

Eagle, W.W. (1958). Elongated styloid process: Symptoms and treatment. *Archives of Otolaryngology*, Vol. 64, pp. 172–176.

Mahan, P., and Alling, C. (1991). *Facial Pain*. Philadelphia: Lea & Febiger, pp. 133–134.

McNamara, J.A., ed. (2000). The Enigma of the Vertical Dimension, monograph 36, Craniofacial Growth Series. University of Michigan: Ann Arbor.

Quiring, D.P., and Warfel, J.H. (1960). *The Head, Neck, and Trunk Muscles and Motor Points*. Philadelphia: Lea & Febiger.

The Effect of Occlusal Forces on the Progression of Periodontal Disease

Stephen K. Harrel, DDS
Martha E. Nunn, DDS, PhD

Occlusal forces on the periodontal supporting structures are routine and normal stresses. Damage to the periodontal structures occurs when occlusal forces exceed the ability of the periodontal structures to resist these forces (Harrel, Nunn, and Hallmon, 2006). The tissue injury that results is referred to as occlusal trauma and is diagnosed at the cellular level. The American Academy of Periodontology 1999 International Workshop for a Classification of Periodontal Diseases and Conditions defined occlusal trauma as "an injury within the attachment apparatus of the dentition when excessive occlusal force(s) exceed the adaptive capability of the affected tissue" (Hallmon, 1999). Occlusal trauma was further defined by the International Workshop as

1. *Primary Occlusal Trauma*—an injury resulting in the periodontal tissue from excessive occlusal forces applied to a tooth or teeth with normal support.
2. *Secondary Occlusal Trauma*—an injury resulting in the periodontal tissue from normal or excessive occlusal forces applied to a tooth or teeth with reduced support.

Because the above definitions of occlusal trauma are based on cellular changes in the tissue that can only be diagnosed in histologic specimens, this chapter will limit itself to the evaluation of the clinical effects of occlusal forces/contacts on the progression of periodontal disease as opposed

Comprehensive Occlusal Concepts in Clinical Practice, by Irwin M. Becker
© 2011 Blackwell Publishing Ltd.

to the cell level effects of occlusal trauma. The term *occlusal trauma* will only be used in reference to publications in the scientific literature that have used the words *occlusal trauma* to describe their findings.

HISTORICAL PERSPECTIVE

Excessive occlusal force has been linked to the progression of periodontal disease for over 100 years (Karolyi, 1901). However, this link has always been controversial, with some groups asserting that specific occlusal forces and certain occlusal contacts are fundamental factors of the periodontal disease process, while others have stated that occlusal forces are not associated with the progression of periodontal disease. An evaluation of this historic controversy is necessary to gain an understanding of the current state of knowledge of the relationship between periodontal disease progression and occlusion.

In the early part of the twentieth century, Stillman set the stage for the controversy surrounding the role of occlusion in the progression of periodontal disease. Stillman stated that trauma from occlusion was the primary cause of periodontal disease and, as such, occlusal treatment was mandatory for the successful treatment and control of periodontal disease (Stillman, 1917, 1926). Stillman believed that all other clinical factors, including oral hygiene and the presence of dental plaque, were secondary to occlusal forces in the pathophysiology of periodontal disease.

AUTOPSY STUDIES

Weinman, in the first half of the twentieth century, questioned Stillman's concepts on occlusion and periodontal disease (Orban and Weinman, 1933; Weinman, 1941; Macapanpan and Weinman, 1954.) Weinmann utilized a series of autopsy specimens to evaluate the progression of inflammation during periodontal destruction. He felt that periodontal inflammation started at the gingival crest and progressed into the supporting structures. Weinman felt that the inflammation progressed in a similar fashion as noted with other surface infections. The progression of the inflammation into the underlying bone followed the course of blood vessels. Weinman did not find any correlation between the occlusal contacts on the teeth and the progression of the periodontal inflammation and bone loss.

In the mid-twentieth century, Glickman reviewed similar autopsy specimens and felt that he saw evidence that occlusal trauma altered the progression of periodontal destruction (Glickman and Smulow, 1962, 1969). Glickman termed the relationship between occlusal trauma and inflammation "co-destruction," and he termed the spread of inflammation in the presence of occlusal trauma an "altered pathway of inflammation." He felt that the progression of inflammation in this altered pathway led to specific patterns of bone loss such as vertical bony defects. Unlike Stillman, Glickman did not feel that occlusal trauma was the initiating cause of periodontal destruction, but he did feel that occlusion was a significant factor in the progression of periodontal disease and that treatment of occlusal trauma was an integral part of the successful control and treatment of periodontal disease.

Following Glickman's publications, Waerhaug also looked at autopsy specimens and found no relationship between occlusal trauma and the progression of periodontal disease (Waerhaug, 1979a, b). Waerhaug could find no evidence for what Glickman had called the altered pathway of inflammation and no evidence that specific bony defects, such as vertical bone loss, were associated with trauma from occlusion. Waerhuag did note that in all cases bacterial plaque was located within 0.5 to 1.5 mm of the connective tissue attachment of the gingiva to the tooth. Waerhuag felt that this association of the "plaque front" to the periodontal attachment apparatus was the sole cause of periodontal inflammation and that occlusal trauma played no part in the progression of periodontal disease.

ANIMAL STUDIES

Because the study of autopsy specimens is observational and therefore subject to evaluator bias, a series of animal studies was performed to try to further elucidate the relationship between occlusion and periodontal disease. Two major animal studies on occlusion were performed by two separate groups of researchers. One group studied the effects of excessive occlusal forces and plaque on squirrel monkeys (Polson, 1974; Polson, Kennedy, and Zander, 1974; Polson, Meitner, and Zander, 1976a, b; Polson and Zander, 1983), and another group studied the same factors in beagle dogs (Lindhe and Svanberg, 1974; Lindhe and Ericsson, 1976; Lindhe and Ericsson, 1982). Both groups found that excessive occlusal forces alone caused loss of bone volume and increased tooth mobility but did not cause attachment loss. From these findings, both groups concluded that occlusal trauma was not an initiating cause of periodontal disease in animals.

When excessive occlusal forces were placed on teeth that had plaque-induced inflammation, the group studying squirrel monkeys again found that there was no loss of periodontal attachment. When excessive occlusal forces were placed on the teeth of beagles that also had plaque-induced inflammation, some loss of attachment was noted. However, this loss of attachment was only noted in the beagle model when surgical reduction of the supporting apparatus had occurred. Both groups concluded that the presence of plaque-induced gingival inflammation was essential to periodontal attachment loss and that excessive occlusal forces were not an initiating factor in periodontal disease in animals. These animal data did not support Stillman's concept that occlusal trauma was the initiating cause of periodontal disease.

Animal studies allowed for the control of many factors that could not be controlled in human studies. These factors include the amount of inflammation allowed to form around the test teeth and the amount of occlusal trauma placed on the teeth. Animal models also allow for the histologic analysis of the effect of various factors on the periodontal supporting apparatus. However, there are several confounders associated with animal studies that make it difficult to transfer the findings in animals to periodontal disease and its treatment in humans. The foremost confounder is the fact that no animal model has naturally occurring periodontal disease similar to that of humans. Another problem is the length of time that the animals were studied. While the animals in these studies were followed for many months, none were followed for the years that are often required for periodontal disease to develop and progress in man. These studies gave great insight into the progression of periodontal disease and the effect of occlusal trauma in animals. The application of these data to humans is problematical.

HUMAN STUDIES

The gold standard for all human clinical studies is the prospective blinded randomized clinical trial. Unfortunately, a randomized clinical trial on the effects of occlusion on the progression of periodontal disease in humans would require the diagnosis of periodontal disease, the diagnosis of occlusal trauma, and then following the patients over time with no treatment of either their periodontal disease or their occlusal trauma. A clinical trial that fulfilled these standards would clearly be unethical in humans as was recognized by the 1996 World Workshop in Periodontics (Proceedings, 1996). Therefore, all studies on the effect of occlusal trauma on the progression of human periodontal disease must rely on studies less powerful than the controlled clinical trial.

Historically, human studies on occlusal trauma have relied on a retrospective analysis of clinical records. These studies have yielded contradictory results, with some studies supporting the supposition that occlusal trauma was a factor in the progression of periodontal disease (Yuodelis and Mann, 1965; Goldstein, 1979; Berhardt et al., 2006) and others showing no relationship between occlusal contacts and the progression of periodontal disease (Shefter and McFall, 1984; Philstrom et al., 1986; Jin and Cao, 1992).

A single human study approached a randomized clinical trial on the effect of occlusal treatment on the outcome of periodontal therapy. Burgett et al. (1992) performed a study where half of a group of patients were randomly selected to receive occlusal adjustment as part of their periodontal therapy and half were not. The patients then received identical periodontal therapy consisting of either nonsurgical or surgical treatment. The patients were then followed over a two-year time period and reevaluated.

The patients who had been assigned to the occlusal adjustment group had a statistically significant improvement in pocket depth when compared with the group that did not receive occlusal therapy. This study appears to give credence to the fact that occlusal adjustment, as part of periodontal therapy, will yield a beneficial effect to periodontal treatment outcomes.

A recent series of studies looked at the effect of occlusal discrepancies on the initial presentation of patients with diagnosed periodontal disease and the effect of either treating or not treating the occlusal discrepancies on the progression of periodontal disease (Nunn and Harrel, 2001, Harrel and Nunn 2001a, b). These studies were unique in the fact that all teeth were evaluated as separate statistical elements rather than evaluating the mean of a patient's pocket depth (patient mean). The patient mean averages the pocket depth of all of the patient's teeth and tends to mask changes that may occur in areas of isolated periodontal destruction. By evaluating each tooth individually, the improvement or worsening of periodontal destruction could be followed on a tooth-by-tooth basis. Also, each *tooth* could be evaluated as having or not having an occlusal discrepancy rather than evaluating each *patient* as having or not having occlusal discrepancies. The individual tooth model was felt to yield an analysis of the role of occlusion on the progression of periodontal disease that is more clinically relevant than studies based on the patient mean.

The outcome of the above-mentioned studies is summarized in figures 7.1 through 7.3. Occlusal discrepancies were designated as a slide between initial contact (centric relation) and maximum intercuspation (centric occlusion) and as a nonworking (balancing) contact. These occlusal discrepancies were associated with deeper pockets at the initial examination than were seen on teeth without these discrepancies. In patients who did not follow through with the recommended treatment, these occlusal discrepancies were associated with a statistically significant greater increase in pocket depths than was found on teeth without the occlusal discrepancies. If occlusal treatment consisting of occlusal adjustment was performed, there was a significant slowing of the increase in pocket depths. In patients who had completed all recommended periodontal treatment, teeth with occlusal discrepancies at the initial evaluation that had undergone occlusal treatment responded as well as teeth without occlusal discrepancies. In patients who had undergone only a part of the periodontal treatment recommended, the progression of periodontal disease as represented by increased pocket depth slowed but continued to progress.

The conclusions drawn from these studies were that the occlusal discrepancies studied represented significant risk factors for the progression of periodontal disease (Harrel, 2003; Hallmon and Harrel, 2004). Teeth that had these occlusal discrepancies were much more likely to present with deeper pockets and, left untreated, were much more likely to have a progression of periodontal disease. Conversely, the treatment of the occlusal discrepancy was associated with a decrease in the risk of forming deeper pockets. Also, with complete periodontal therapy, including surgery where

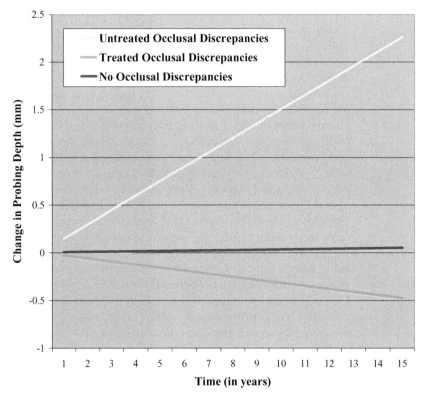

Fig. 7.1. Change in probing depth (tooth-based data) over time. Includes patients who completed all recommended periodontal treatment (control group), patients who self-selected not to have treatment (untreated group), and patients who completed nonsurgical therapy but not the recommended surgical treatment (partially treated group). Adapted from Harrel and Nunn, 2001a. Reprinted with permission from the American Academy of Periodontology.

indicated, teeth with initial occlusal discrepancies no longer demonstrated a higher risk factor for deeper pockets and were associated with a positive clinical outcome from periodontal therapy.

Another study of the same group of patients as above showed that other occlusal contacts contributed in a similar manner to deeper pockets as the two occlusal discrepancies originally reported on. The findings of this study are summarized in figures 7.4 through 7.7. This study confirmed that premature contacts in centric relation and nonworking contacts were significant risk factors for deeper periodontal pockets (Harrel and Nunn, 2009). It also showed that the greater the discrepancy between centric relation and centric occlusion, that is, the greater the length of "slide," the greater the risk for deeper pockets. This was true for vertical, horizontal, and lateral movements. The greater the length of slide, the greater was the risk for deeper pockets. Additionally, teeth with combined working and

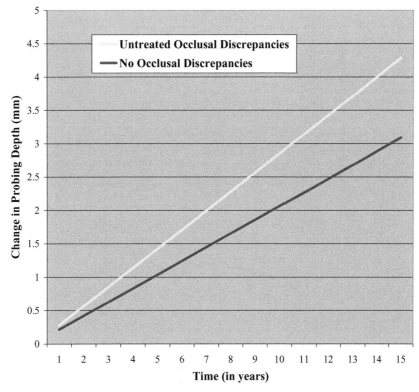

Fig. 7.2. Change in probing depth (tooth-based data) over time for patients diagnosed with periodontal disease who self-selected to not receive periodontal treatment (untreated group). Adapted from Harrel and Nunn, 2001a. Reprinted with permission from the American Academy of Periodontology.

balancing contacts ("cross-tooth balance") and posterior teeth with protrusive contacts were at greater risk for deeper pockets. Interestingly, anterior teeth with protrusive contacts were at less risk for deeper pockets than anterior teeth that did not have a protrusive contact. In all cases of various contacts being a significant risk factor for deeper pockets, the risk represented by the occlusal contacts was between two and four times greater than the risk inherent in the traditional periodontal risk factors of smoking, male gender, and unsatisfactory oral hygiene.

When the presence of recession was evaluated, no negative relationship was found between the width of keratinized gingiva and centric premature contacts or nonworking contacts (Harrel and Nunn, 2004). This was also true for teeth with combined balancing and working contacts, as well as posterior teeth with protrusive contacts. Interestingly, there was an increased width of keratinized gingiva, that is, a positive statistical relationship, on anterior teeth with protrusive contacts (Harrel and Nunn,

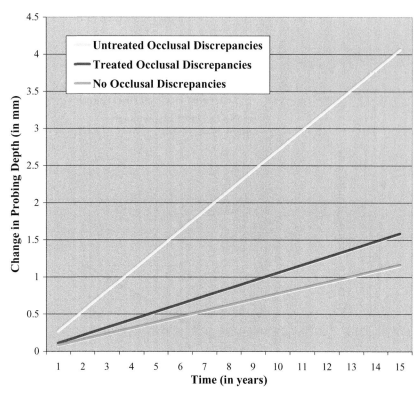

Fig. 7.3. Change in probing depth (tooth-based data) over time for patients who completed nonsurgical treatment but not the recommended surgical treatment (partially treated group). Adapted from Harrel and Nunn, 2001a. Reprinted with permission from the American Academy of Periodontology.

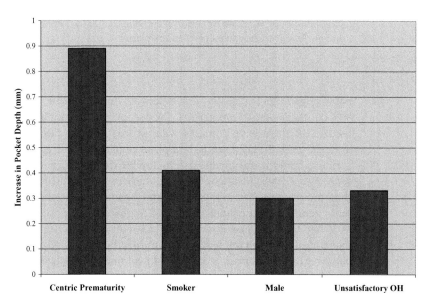

Fig. 7.4. Increase in probing depth of teeth with a centric prematurity compared to traditional risk factors related to increased probing depth (OH = oral hygiene). Adapted from Harrel and Nunn, 2009.

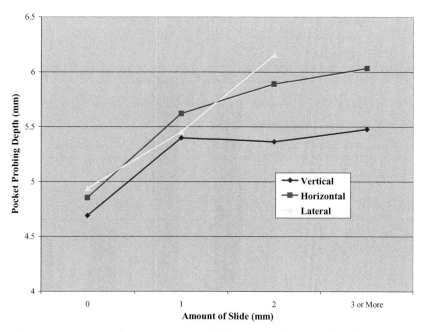

Fig. 7.5. Association between amount of slide (vertical, horizontal, and lateral) and pocket probing depth (tooth-based data).

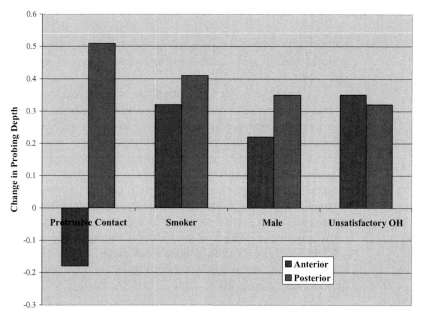

Fig. 7.6. Change in probing depth of teeth with contact in protrusive movement by tooth position (anterior versus posterior) compared to traditional risk factors related to increased probing depth.

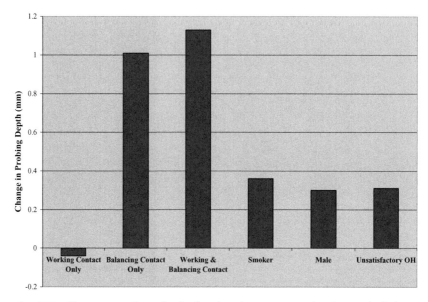

Fig. 7.7. Change in probing depth of teeth with contact type (working only, balancing only, working and balancing) compared to traditional risk factors related to increased probing depth. Adapted from Harrel and Nunn, 2009.

2009). These findings run counter to the clinical assumption that excessive occlusal forces can cause a reduction in gingival width and lead to recession.

The current status of the relationship between occlusion and periodontal disease remains controversial despite the findings of recent research. The views of many educators appear to be strongly influenced by the animal studies published up to thirty years ago, and the treatment of occlusal discrepancies is not routinely emphasized in the treatment of periodontal disease. Current human research does not support many of the findings from past animal research, but the de-emphasis of occlusal treatment in the treatment of periodontal disease persists. This approach is currently being reassessed due to recent research, but occlusion treatment remains a portion of periodontal therapy that may not be given adequate attention in the education of general dentists or periodontists. This may translate to inadequate treatment of a significant risk factor for periodontal destruction.

OCCLUSAL FINDINGS AS A PART OF PERIODONTAL DIAGNOSIS

A basic analysis of occlusal contacts should be an integral part of all periodontal examinations. This analysis does not have to be in detail but should allow the examiner to determine if the patient's occlusion is a factor in his or her periodontal condition and whether occlusal therapy should be part of the patient's periodontal treatment. The patient should be placed in a retruded position and asked to close until first contact. This contact or contacts should be evaluated and recorded. The amount and direction of movement between a retruded (centric) position and maximum intercuspation should be recorded. From a point of maximum intercuspation, contacts in working, nonworking, and protrusive contacts should be recorded. Finding these contacts can be done by direct visualization or the use of marking ribbon.

The use of mounted models may be beneficial but is usually not necessary at the initial examination appointment. The goal of this initial evaluation is to gain a working knowledge of the patient's occlusal relationship to assist in periodontal treatment planning. Detailed information on occlusal relationships can be obtained utilizing a variety of methods if treatment of the occlusion is deemed necessary.

OCCLUSION AS A FACTOR IN TREATMENT PLANNING OF PERIODONTAL THERAPY

The typical periodontal patient may present with multiple dental concerns, but his or her periodontal condition and the outcome of periodontal therapy will often dictate how the other dental concerns are addressed. Part of periodontal treatment planning will be the assignment of prognosis for each tooth. The periodontal prognosis will determine which teeth cannot be treated and will be extracted (hopeless prognosis), which teeth will be salvageable with periodontal therapy (good to fair prognosis), and which teeth may or may not be salvageable with periodontal treatment (questionable prognosis). It is not uncommon for the prognosis of a tooth to change during initial nonsurgical treatment. Because of this initial uncertainty concerning the long-term prognosis of individual teeth, it is frequently necessary to perform nonsurgical periodontal treatment to ameliorate periodontal inflammation, mobility, and other factors. Often the patient is reevaluated several weeks to several months after this initial therapy before a definitive diagnosis is assigned to individual teeth.

Because of the initial uncertainty of the prognosis of each individual tooth, the role of occlusal treatment planning and therapy during periodontal therapy is often very different than in other disciplines of dentistry. When occlusion is evaluated as part of an orthodontic treatment plan, a projection can be made about the ability to move the teeth and occlusal surfaces toward an idealized occlusal relationship. This may include changing the skeletal relationship of the jaws and altering the alignment of each individual tooth. Likewise, restorative treatment can significantly alter occlusion toward a more ideal relationship by changing the occlusal anatomy and possibly changing the tooth's angulation by manipulating the fabrication of the restorations.

Because of the uncertainty of the final periodontal prognosis of individual teeth and possibly entire arches, periodontal therapy has to alter existing occlusal relationship without the advantage of being able to change the position of teeth, the angulation of crowns, or extensively changing the occlusal anatomy of teeth. Instead, occlusal therapy for periodontal patients must initially be confined to the alteration of natural teeth and restorations as they exist (selective grinding) and/or the fabrication of removable occlusal appliances. The long-term treatment plan for periodontal patients may well include orthodontic and/or extensive prosthetic therapy aimed at establishing a more ideal occlusion, but this more ideal relationship is often not possible until a final prognosis and periodontal health have been established.

OCCLUSAL THERAPY FOR THE PERIODONTAL PATIENT— TEETH WITH A POOR PROGNOSIS

As is the case in all aspects of periodontal therapy, the projected long-term prognosis of the tooth or arch should be considered when performing occlusal therapy for the periodontal patient. If an entire arch is considered to have a poor or questionable prognosis, the use of a removable appliance may be the best approach for treating occlusion. As an example, if a full denture or overdenture is planned for the maxilla, then a maxillary removable appliance that covers and stabilizes all of the maxillary teeth will probably allow for greater patient comfort and function while periodontal therapy is performed on the mandibular teeth and a definitive prosthesis for the maxilla is fabricated. If only a single tooth has a hopeless prognosis but will be retained until a later stage of therapy, it may be advantageous for comfort and function to perform selective grinding that takes that tooth out of all occlusal contact. This tooth will eventually erupt back into an occlusal relationship, but it will probably be extracted before this becomes a treatment concern.

OCCLUSAL THERAPY FOR THE PERIODONTAL PATIENT— TEETH TO BE RETAINED

If occlusal contacts that have been established as risk factors for the progression of periodontal disease exist in a patient with periodontal disease, occlusal therapy should be a part of definitive periodontal treatment. Selective grinding should be performed on teeth that are projected to be retained long-term and/or removable occlusal appliances should be fabricated. As noted previously, an idealized occlusal relation endpoint is often not possible during the initial stages of periodontal therapy. The goal of occlusal therapy during initial periodontal treatment should be to minimize the number of damaging contacts that are present on the teeth. Specifically, to the greatest extent possible, premature contacts in centric relation and slides to centric occlusion should be minimized. Nonworking contacts (balancing) should be minimized and protrusive contacts on posterior teeth should be relieved. Fremitus, mobility of the teeth during function, should be relieved to the greatest extent possible. Fremitus is often associated with a tooth having both working and balancing contacts (cross-tooth balance).

When completed, the above noted damaging contacts will have been removed to the greatest extent possible and bilateral contact on the existing dentition will have been made as even as possible. This end result may well be far removed from an idealized occlusal relationship with bilateral contacts and even pressure on both sides, no nonworking contacts, and a cuspid-protected occlusion. This more idealized occlusal relationship must be delayed until after the periodontal disease has been successfully treated and the teeth stabilized.

OCCLUSAL THERAPY FOR THE PERIODONTAL PATIENT— REMOVABLE APPLIANCES

Removable appliances have many applications in the treatment and alterations of occlusal relationships. These include the stabilization of mobile teeth, positioning of the jaws, treatment for parafunctional habits, and many other uses. The removable appliance has the advantage that all changes to the occlusion can be reversed by the removal of the appliance. Because of this inherent advantage, a removable appliance is often recommended as the first step in occlusal therapy before procedures such as selective grinding are performed.

Removable appliances also have an inherent and major disadvantage in the fact that they only affect the occlusion and periodontal health while the patient is wearing them. If the patient is not compliant with treatment recommendations, minimal improvement will be noted with the use of a removable appliance. Because of this disadvantage, selective grinding of the natural dentition is the preferred method for treating occlusal discrepancies associated with periodontal disease progression. The use of removable appliances during periodontal therapy is often limited to the treatment of parafunctional habits.

The special needs of the periodontal patient should be considered during design of the removable occlusal appliance. Because periodontal patients generally have a weakened periodontal support apparatus, an appliance should be fabricated that will stabilize the occlusion and not place excessive stress and pressures on teeth with a weakened support. An example would be a patient with periodontal disease on the maxillary anteriors and bicuspids. It is likely that the fabrication of a mandibular removable appliance should be avoided for this patient.

The very nature of a mandibular appliance tends to place some amount of wedging pressure on the maxillary anterior teeth. When the maxillary anterior teeth are healthy, they will usually resist this wedging pressure. However, with maxillary teeth that are periodontally weakened, this wedging pressure will tend to increase mobility and force these teeth into an anterior flared position. While a mandibular appliance may be acceptable or even desirable for a patient with a healthy dentition, this same appliance may be detrimental to the periodontal patient. Within this same context, the use of an appliance with built-in cuspid disclusion or an anterior disclusion ramp may also be detrimental if the periodontal patient has weakened cuspids or anterior teeth.

As with treatment planning and use of selective grinding for the periodontal patient, the design of removable appliances needs to take into consideration the special risks of the periodontal patient. In most cases during periodontal treatment, the use of a maxillary appliance with a flat group function occlusion is usually best during active periodontal treatment. If positioning appliances or appliances with a specific type of disclusion pattern are needed for the long-term maintenance of the patient or to accomplish a specific treatment goal, these appliances should be fabricated after the periodontal condition has been stabilized and periodontal health has been established.

PERIODONTAL MAINTENANCE

The long-term success of periodontal therapy depends on ongoing periodontal maintenance care. This usually entails frequent routine cleaning of the teeth and reinforcement of oral hygiene procedures. As part of periodontal maintenance, the occlusion should be reevaluated at all visits. Occlusal relationships are never static and will change with wear, restorations, and other factors. Because of generally reduced periodontal support in patients with past periodontal disease, the occlusion of periodontal patients may be more prone to change than that of a periodontally healthy patient. Due to this, occlusal relationships should be monitored closely and minor occlusal adjustments may be necessary as part of a periodontal maintenance program.

SUMMARY

Occlusal forces have been closely linked with the progression of periodontal disease. While this relationship has been controversial for many years, recent human study seems to confirm that certain occlusal contacts are significant risk factors for periodontal destruction. All patients who have periodontal disease should have their occlusion evaluated as part of a complete periodontal examination, and the findings from this occlusal evaluation should be incorporated into the treatment planning for the patient. Where indicated, occlusal treatment, consisting of selective grinding, is indicated to eliminate occlusal contacts that have been shown to be risk factors for periodontal disease. Removable occlusal appliances can also be a part of this occlusal treatment. Definitive occlusal therapy such as prosthetic occlusal rehabilitation and/or orthodontic therapy should not be performed until the patient's periodontal condition has been treated and the teeth are periodontally stable. Occlusal contacts should be routinely monitored as part of a periodontal maintenance program.

REFERENCES

Berhardt, O., et al. (2006). The influence of dynamic occlusal interferences on probing depth and attachment level: Result of the study of health in Pomerania (SHIP). *Journal of Periodontology*, Vol. 77, pp. 506–516.

Burgett, F., Ramfjord, S., Nissle, R., et al. (1992). A randomized trial of occlusal adjustment in the treatment of periodontitis patients. *Journal of Clinical Periodontology*, Vol. 19, pp. 381–387.

Glickman, I., and Smulow, J.B. (1962). Alterations in the pathway of gingival inflammation into the underlying tissues induced by excessive occlusal forces. *Journal of Periodontology*, Vol. 33, pp. 7–13.

Glickman, I., and Smulow, J. (1969). The combined effects of inflammation and trauma from occlusion in periodontitis. *International Dental Journal*, Vol. 39, pp. 101–105.

Goldstein, G.R. (1979). The relationship of canine-protected occlusion to a periodontal index. *Journal of Prosthetic Dentistry*, Vol. 41, pp. 277–283.

Hallmon, W.W. (1999). Occlusal trauma: Effect and impact on the periodontium. Consensus report: Occlusal trauma. American Academy of Periodontology, 1999 International Workshop for a Classification of Periodontal Diseases and Conditions. *Annals of Periodontology*, Vol. 1, pp. 102–108.

Hallmon, W.W., and Harrel, S.K. (2004). Occlusal analysis, diagnosis and management in the practice of periodontics. *Periodontology 2000*, Vol. 34, pp. 151–164.

Harrel, S.K. (2003). Occlusal forces as a risk factor for periodontal disease. *Periodontology 2000*, Vol. 32, pp. 111–117.

Harrel, S.K., and Nunn, M.E. (2001a). The effect of occlusal discrepancies on treated and untreated periodontitis: II. Relationship of occlusal treatment to the progression of periodontal disease. *Journal of Periodontology*, Vol. 72, pp. 495–505.

Harrel, S.K., and Nunn, M.E. (2001b). Longitudinal comparison of the periodontal status of patients with moderate to severe periodontal disease receiving no treatment, non-surgical treatment, and surgical treatment utilizing individual sites for analysis. *Journal of Periodontology* 2001, Vol. 72, pp. 1509–1519.

Harrel, S.K., and Nunn, M.E. (2004). The effect of occlusal discrepancies on gingival width. *Journal of Periodontology*, Vol. 75, pp. 98–105.

Harrel, S.K., and Nunn, M.E. (2009). The association of occlusal contacts with the presence of increased periodontal probing depth. *Journal of Clinical Periodontology*, Vol. 36, pp. 1035–1042.

Harrel, S.K., Nunn, M.E., and Hallmon, W.W. (2006). Is there an association between occlusion and periodontal destruction? Yes—Occlusal forces can contribute to periodontal destruction. *Journal of the American Dental Association*, Vol. 137, pp. 1380–1392.

Jin, L., and Cao, C. (1992). Clinical diagnosis of trauma from occlusion and its relation with severity of periodontitis. *Journal of Clinical Periodontology*, Vol. 19, pp. 92–97.

Karolyi, M. (1901). Beobachtungen über pyorrhea alveolaris. *Öst. Ung. Vierteeljschr Zahnheilk*, Vol. 17, p. 279.

Lindhe, J., and Ericsson, I. (1976). Influence of trauma from occlusion on reduced but healthy periodontal tissues in dogs. *Journal of Clinical Periodontology*, Vol. 3, pp. 110–122.

Lindhe, J., and Ericsson, I. (1982). The effect of elimination of jiggling forces on periodontally exposed teeth in the dog. *Journal of Periodontology*, Vol. 53, pp. 562–567.

Lindhe, J., and Svanberg, G. (1974). Influence of trauma from occlusion on the progression of experimental periodontitis in the beagle dog. *Journal of Clinical Periodontology*, Vol. 1, pp. 3–14.

Macapanpan, L.C., and Weinman J. (1954). The influence of injury to the periodontal membrane on the spread of gingival inflammation. *Journal of Dental Research*, Vol. 33, pp. 263–272.

Nunn, M., and Harrel, S.K. (2001). The effect of occlusal discrepancies on treated and untreated periodontitis: I. Relationship of initial occlusal discrepancies to initial clinical parameters. *Journal of Periodontology*, Vol. 72, pp. 485–494.

Orban, B., and Weinman, J. (1933). Signs of traumatic occlusion in average human jaws. *Journal of Dental Research*, Vol. 13, pp. 216.

Philstrom, P.B., Anderson, K., Aeppli, D., et al. (1986). Association between signs of trauma from occlusion and periodontitis. *Journal of Periodontology*, Vol. 57, pp. 1–6.

Polson, A. (1974). Trauma and progression of marginal periodontitis in squirrel monkeys: II. Co-destructive factors of periodontitis and mechanically produced injury. *Journal of Periodontal Research*, Vol. 9, pp. 108–113.

Polson, A., Kennedy, J., and Zander, H. (1974). Trauma and progression of periodontitis in squirrel monkeys: I. Co-destructive factors of periodontitis and thermally produced injury. *Journal of Periodontal Research*, Vol. 9, pp. 100–107.

Polson, A., Meitner, S., and Zander, H. (1976a). Trauma and progression of marginal periodontitis in squirrel monkeys: III. Adaptation of interproximal alveolar bone to repetitive injury. *Journal of Periodontal Research*, Vol. 11, pp. 179–289.

Polson, A., Meitner, S., and Zander, H. (1976b). Trauma and progression of marginal periodontitis in squirrel monkeys: IV. Reversibility of bone loss due to trauma alone and trauma superimposed upon periodontitis. *Journal of Periodontal Research*, Vol. 11, pp. 290–297.

Polson, A., and Zander, H. (1983). Effects of periodontal trauma on intrabony pockets. *Journal of Periodontology*, Vol. 54, pp. 586–591.

Proceedings of the 1996 World Workshop in Periodontics. Lansdowne, Virginia, July 13-17. *Annals of Periodontology*, Vol. 1, pp. 1–947.

Proceedings of the 1999 International Workshop for a Classification of Periodontal Diseases and Conditions. Oak Brook, Illinois, October 30–November 2. *Annals of Periodontology*, Vol. 4, pp. 1–112.

Shefter, G., and McFall, W. (1984). Occlusal relations and periodontal status in human adults. *Journal of Periodontology*, Vol. 55, pp. 368–374.

Stillman, P.R. (1917). The management of pyorrhea. *Dental Cosmos*, Vol. 59, pp. 405–414.

Stillman, P.R. (1926). What is traumatic occlusion and how can it be diagnosed and corrected? *Journal of the American Dental Association*, Vol. 12, pp. 1330–1338.

Waerhaug, J. (1979a). The angular bone defect and its relationship to trauma from occlusion and downgrowth of subgingival plaque. *Journal of Clinical Periodontology*, Vol. 6, pp. 61–82.

Waerhaug, J. (1979b). The infrabony pocket and its relationship to trauma from occlusion and subgingival plaque. *Journal of Periodontology*, Vol. 50, pp. 355–365.

Weinman, J. (1941). Progress of gingival inflammation into the supporting structure of the teeth. *Journal of Periodontology*, Vol. 12, pp. 71–76.

Yuodelis, R.A., and Mann, W.V. (1965). The prevalence of and possible role of non-working contacts in periodontal disease. *Periodontics*, Vol. 3, pp. 219–223.

An Occlusal Basis of Treatment Planning

Irwin M. Becker, DDS

Perhaps the real genius of the Pankey-Mann-Schuyler methodology (Mann and Pankey, 1960; Schuyler, 1961) can be found in its simplification and clarification of how to piece together the puzzle of treatment planning. It has evolved today into a rationale, protocol, and method of analyzing the various parts of the stomatognathic system and then determining a straightforward way of treatment planning almost any case, no matter how complicated.

Schuyler (2001) lists the five basic required factors that influence immediate posterior disclusion:

- Condylar inclination
- Anterior guidance
- Plane of occlusion
- Axial inclination of each tooth
- Cusp-fossa inclination of the posterior teeth

CONDYLAR INCLINATION

Since the earliest use of articulators, face bows, and other apparatuses, dentists and researchers have tried to create a machine that replicates the exact condylar inclination. At one point, there was an articulator with two condylar heads that could replicate both the protrusive inclination and the balancing side inclination, which are normally not the same. Thus, any time one set condylar inclination, say with a protrusive check bite, there

Comprehensive Occlusal Concepts in Clinical Practice, by Irwin M. Becker
© 2011 Blackwell Publishing Ltd.

could be some inherent error. For example, when one makes a protrusive record and the patient is asked to close edge to edge in protrusive movement, if the wax has some degree of hardness, it could dislodge the condyle from its position on the eminence, creating a significant error.

Most condylar movements down the slope of the eminence are quite curvilinear. Wherever movement is stopped to make the protrusive record, the record is being made at some point on this magnificent curvilinear slope. The slope is not a straight line representing a specific angle. So what does the condylar angle number mean?

Zero almost always represents the placement parallel to the position used to record the face bow. Some articulator systems utilize the Frankfort horizontal plane. Others utilize the Camper's line, and still others use the nasion or infraorbital foramen. Thus, the number listed is only a reference point compared to the zero of how the face bow was set up.

The average angle of inclination in a normal, healthy individual is around 45 to 50 degrees. The practitioner does not really need to know the exact number but does want to know if the inclination is steep, normal, or shallow. This helps the practitioner assess the amount of help the condylar inclination provides in movement to posterior disclusion.

The Pankey Institute instructs practitioners in the use of the protrusive record and also in making direct observations in the mouth prior to setting an inclination on the articulator that mimics what is observed in the mouth. The practitioner customizes the condylar inclination of the articulator by matching the observed amount of either balancing or protrusive separation of the teeth. Figures 8.1 to 8.7 clearly demonstrate this technique, which

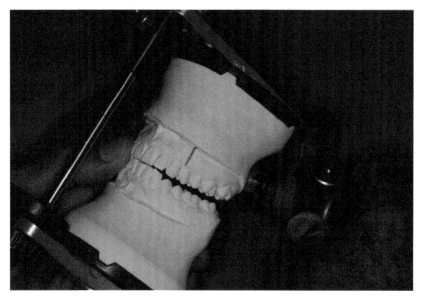

Fig. 8.1. Dialing in a steep condylar inclination (note the excessive balancing side separation).

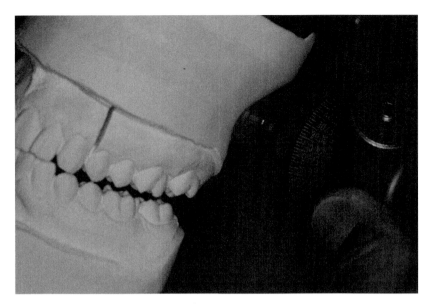

Fig. 8.2. Dialing in a moderate inclination.

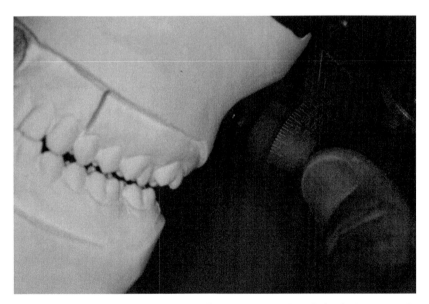

Fig. 8.3. Dialing in a shallow inclination (note the slight balancing side separation).

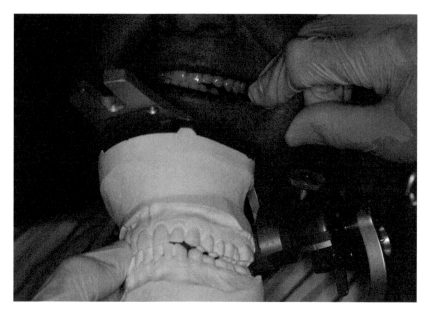

Fig. 8.4. Checking with chairside observations that amount of disclusion is similar both intraorally and on the articulator.

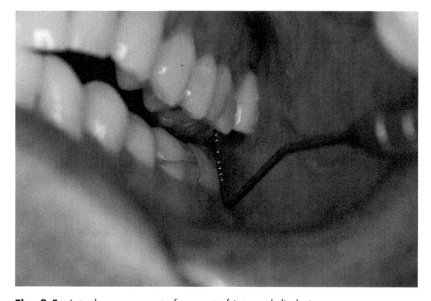

Fig. 8.5. Actual measurement of amount of intraoral disclusion.

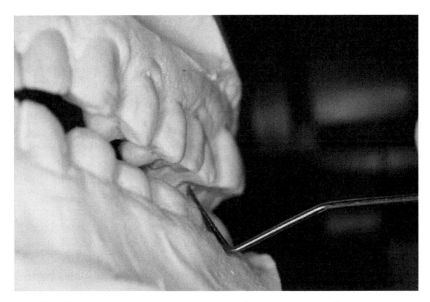

Fig. 8.6. Dialing in a condylar setting to match exact posterior disclusion.

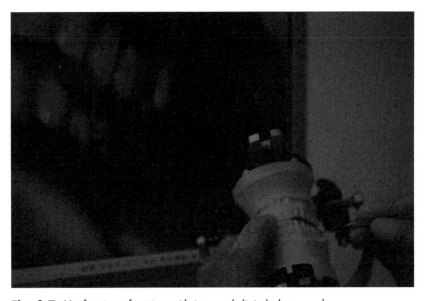

Fig. 8.7. Verification of setting with intraoral digital photograph.

can be accomplished during the exam or at a later appointment after the casts have been mounted. Simply record the amount of separation or lack thereof by digital photography or direct measurement with a periodontal probe.

Another way to make sure the articulator settings are correct is by matching wear patterns. If there are definitive wear patterns in any excursive movement, they should actually touch on the articulated study casts. If they do not, a shallower inclination should be dialed so they do touch.

Anterior crossover patterns should also match on the articulated casts, exactly as seen intraorally. It is important to understand that as inclination is made steeper on the articulator, the balancing side teeth are not only separated but the entire maxilla is shifted. This directly affects how the anterior teeth appear to line up against each other. Figures 8.8 to 8.10 demonstrate this phenomenon.

For years, it was common practice to set the condylar inclination at an average setting, such as 20 degrees. This was done to ensure the articulator was less steep than the mouth. When the technician made restorations, he or she made sure the anterior teeth cleared on the articulator. Because the mouth was steeper, a balancing interference was not inadvertently created. That practice worked well to address balancing or protrusive interferences on the working casts but did not address other circumstances.

Today almost all cases get preoperative diagnostic workups, and the objective should be to have the casts functioning on the articulator just as

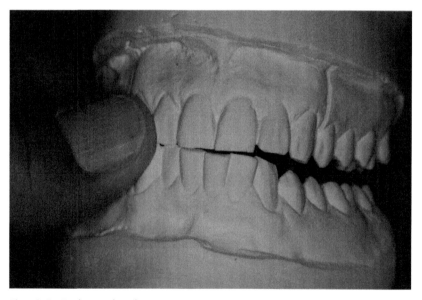

Fig. 8.8. Dialing in by observing crossover wear patterns—too steep.

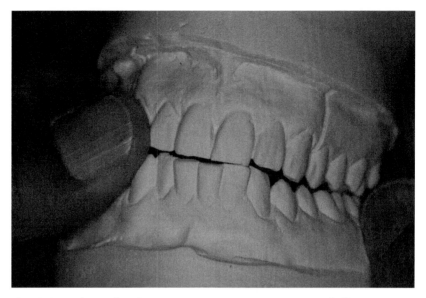

Fig. 8.9. Dialing in by observing crossover wear patterns—too shallow.

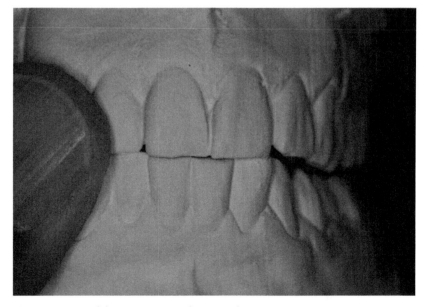

Fig. 8.10. Condylar setting just right to match crossover wear pattern.

the teeth do in the mouth. Modeling actual function is important as the practitioner makes decisions about equilibration, crossover relationships, and specific anterior guidance details on both the bite splint setup and the actual anterior wax-up.

ANTERIOR GUIDANCE

Each of the five factors listed above plays a positive or negative role in helping posterior teeth to disclude. Except for condylar inclination (a given), each of the other factors can be manipulated, changed, or left alone. It is important to know the approximate steepness of the condylar inclination in order to judge if the case is a tight tolerance case. If there is not much disclusive help from the steepness of the eminence, then help will be needed from other of the four factors. Not much posterior lift can be achieved when the patient has a degenerative or arthritic condylar condition (Dawson, 1973; Kirveskarari, Alanen, and Jamsa, 1989).

A close look at the other four factors reveals situations that the clinician can work with on a daily basis. Anterior guidance, for example, can be steepened if needed, but only to a degree. The safest way to deal with this factor is to utilize the shallowest inclines that still disclude the posterior teeth. When attempting to go beyond this level of anterior steepness, the practitioner often inadvertently invades or violates the envelope of function (Schuyler, 2001).

When the envelope of function is invaded, the patient reports a tight, uncomfortable feeling in the anterior region. Chewing becomes difficult and the patient reports that the upper and lower front teeth sometimes bang into each other. Sometimes speech is affected. Figure 8.11 demon-

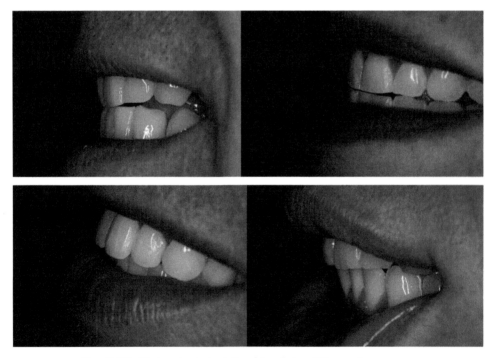

Fig. 8.11. Various incisal relationships during "S" sounds.

strates the one square inch typically needed for proper "s" sounds. When the anterior steepness violates the chewing envelope, speech is often negatively affected, whether the one square inch space occurs at the edge-to-edge position or toward the cingulum of the upper lingual surface.

Today, esthetic considerations play a role in deciding which tooth is shortened to treat interferences. Chapter 11 discusses this in detail (Spear, 2002).

ENVELOPE OF PARAFUNCTION

A further discussion is needed to describe the issue of attempting to restore anterior teeth to a position or steepness that violates the patient's "envelope of parafunction." This is a new term that can help clinicians better understand the complex problem of restoring anterior teeth to beauty, form, and function.

When adding length and steepness to restore a youthful appearance, the practitioner commonly produces a plane similar to that of patients who have worn the same teeth down due to a parafunctional habit. Chapter 11 describes the details of restorative dentistry that will enable the reader to more predictably make decisions based on violations of the envelope of parafunction.

It is sufficient to recognize at this point that patterns of wear and destruction already occur and to understand the nature of these patterns. If they appear to be laterally induced and formed during lateral parafunctional movements, then adding steepness is counterproductive to long-lasting results. If there are no lateral patterns of wear or there exist indications of a vertical pattern, then increasing steepness may be more than appropriate.

It seems that some patients can adapt to increased steepness and others have disastrous sequelae. It is the obligation of the clinician to find out during provisional or mocked-up bonded transitional restorations whether this patient is adaptable or not. Preexisting wear patterns can tell the practitioner a lot about the lack of adaptability. Once the patient has demonstrated the ability to wear down tooth enamel, it is likely the patient could wear down chrome bumper.

PLANE OF OCCLUSION

Just like orthodontists have been taught, a flat plane of occlusion is easier to disclude and can get by with a shallower anterior guidance. When there is a steep curve of Spee or Wilson, difficult disclusion is likely, especially in protrusive. Thus, in a tight tolerance case, where there is little separation from both condylar guidance and anterior guidance, there is no choice but to utilize a shallow plane of occlusion.

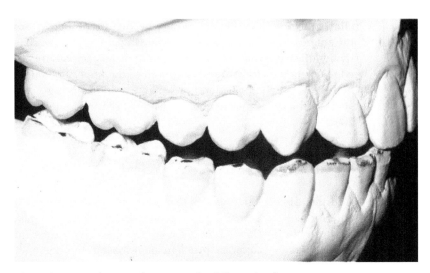

Fig. 8.12. Violation of curve of Wilson leading to posterior crossover interference.

The practitioner must also consider esthetics. Functionally, the only real issue relating to plane of occlusion is whether immediate posterior disclusion can be achieved. Although it may be acceptable occlusally to have a two-step plane when there has been supereruption of the lower anterior section, as evidenced by a change in the gingival margin (bone and tissue came with the dental unit), this type of plane may not have a pleasing appearance.

When there is a violation of curve of Wilson, a posterior crossover, parafunctional type of interferences may be observed. Figure 8.12 demonstrates this type of common problem. When the lower lingual cusps are higher than their corresponding buccal cusps, the author's preference is to reduce the lingual height. This is a strong indication for an orthodontic evaluation or at least a diagnostic workup to determine the possibility of organizing the occlusion (equilibration).

AXIAL INCLINATION OF EACH TOOTH

Perhaps the very best rationale for up righting inclined teeth is to improve the ability to achieve disclusion. As a given posterior tooth begins to collapse forward (mesial vector of force), the distal aspect rapidly becomes a protrusive interference. Also, it is critical to attempt to have the patient vertically loaded at each tooth contact. An inclined tooth is not axially loaded. Therefore, it is imperative that the clinician discuss these important issues with each patient so the patient can make an informed health decision.

It is not uncommon for the dentist to err in deciding not to mention orthodontics under the assumption that the patient will not accept orthodontic therapy. A very important characteristic of the "comprehensive dentist" is not creating a treatment plan based on what he or she thinks the patient will accept. It is much more important to discuss all appropriate options and then figure out with the patient how to accomplish an optimal therapeutic treatment plan.

CUSP-FOSSA INCLINATION

For many decades the debate has raged in the literature over whether sharper or flat teeth function better. In complete denture prosthodontics, it has been shown that immediate posterior disclusion is not needed to reduce muscle activity due to the lack of periodontal ligament proprioceptors. Therefore, it becomes a clinician's choice.

However, in natural or restored dentitions, the problem of immediate disclusion must be considered. When it is a tight tolerance case (lack of anterior guidance or condylar inclination), a flatter morphology is preferable. The author has observed that patients do quite well with a flatter anatomy and disclusion is made much easier. Patient age and presenting condition may come into play. In cases where there is no wear or mobility, patients may be able to keep their more youthful anatomy. In implant cases or cases with advanced periodontal disease, the author prefers to keep the patients in flatter anatomy.

THE OCCLUSAL TREATMENT PLANNING CHECKLIST

The author uses the following list during occlusal treatment planning for each comprehensive exam patient.

- Diagnosis of pain, infection and/or inflammation—perio-endo considerations
- Esthetic considerations
- Parafunctional considerations
- Orthodontic-orthognathic considerations
- Restorative-occlusal considerations

This checklist is helpful when doing phase 1 analysis prior to more definitive aspects of dentistry and provides a systematic path for thinking about all items uncovered during the codiscovery exam. The reader should remember that this text is focused on occlusal issues. In comprehensive treatment planning, *all* issues would be reviewed at this point. The checklist would be expanded to include all periodontal concerns, medical issues, all soft tissue and hard tissue pathologies, any possible neurological and hematological issues, and certainly any structural issues of the stomatognathic system (Amsterdam, 1974). Also, the status of the joint condition would have to be assessed in detail before proceeding with treatment planning decisions.

DIAGNOSTIC TREE

Figure 8.13 illustrates a diagnostic thought process used for years by the author to take the mound of information gathered during a codiscovery exam and pour it into a manageable diagnostic funnel from which the basic treatment plan will evolve. It is NOT a shortcut in the comprehensive exam but rather a simplified means of identifying the most important sets of data.

If the clinician can summarize the data from the five most critical elements of the occlusal exam, then it becomes a more manageable process to create an appropriate diagnosis (Dawson, 1999). Therefore, muscle palpation, load testing, history, joint auscultation, and occlusal findings will guide the astute clinician into not only a written diagnosis but also the ability to draw a basic stick drawing that describes the essential structures of the joint. This drawing becomes a helpful tool for patient education as well as formulation of a clear diagnosis.

Figures 8.14 and 8.15 illustrate a displaced disc and then a total loss of disc with subsequent degenerative destruction of articulating surface.

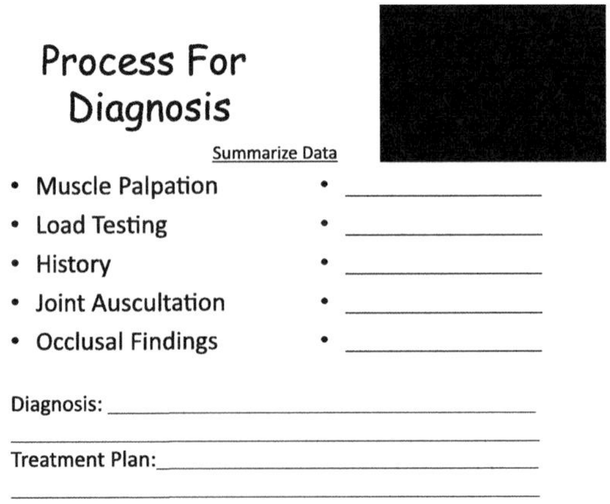

Fig. 8.13. Diagnostic tree.

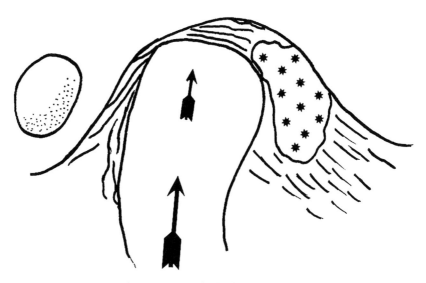

Fig. 8.14. Diagram indicating anteriorly displaced disc. Courtesy of Rick Gonzalez.

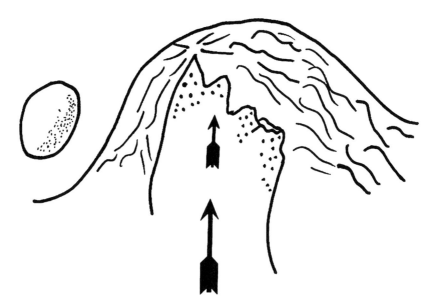

Fig. 8.15. Diagram demonstrating degenerative or arthritic destruction of condyle. Courtesy of Rick Gonzalez.

PIECING THE TREATMENT PLANNING PUZZLE TOGETHER

Treatment planning usually starts with solving the anterior guidance question and then addressing any plane of occlusion issues. If the clinician looks at each part as a piece of a puzzle, the solution appears like a

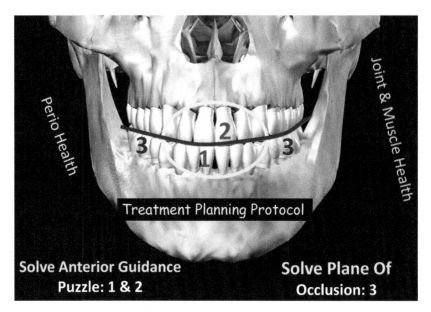

Fig. 8.16. The treatment planning sequence.

cookbook recipe. As each piece of the puzzle is evaluated, the practitioner may find treatment is not needed for every piece.

The practitioner should think through appropriate treatment that is least aggressive or invasive. Perhaps one of the most important approaches that Dr. L.D. Pankey came up with was "asking the question of what needs to be done, if anything, that brings each of the pieces to optimal health, comfort, function and beauty" (Mann and Pankey, 1960). That question should guide most treatment decisions even today.

Figure 8.16 is a clever reminder of the classic PMS methodology of treatment planning and often sequencing of treatment. If the clinician follows these steps and answers Pankey's question above, the answer will become obvious, especially if a meaningful and impactful new patient experience has been previously accomplished.

The methodology shown above will enable the reader to evaluate almost any patient situation with confidence for beginning a sensible and well thought-out treatment sequence, by piecing the pieces together in the suggested order. Please note that when the clinician is examining chairside, the maxillary anterior teeth are often placed in step I, but once the casts are articulated, the clinician generally places the lower anterior incisal plane into step I. The correct placement and correction of this plane (if change is needed) will get the clinician started and help make critical determinations such as vertical dimension. Once a reasonable anterior guidance is worked out on the casts, the overall plane of occlusion can be addressed. Again, it can be changed, if needed, or it can be left alone. The techniques used to make these changes are based on clinical judgment and personal preferences. Note that the "least invasive" often comes into play, as long as the appropriate objectives can be obtained.

It is critical to remember that even though this text is consumed with the principles of occlusion, often the most important first step is to obtain and plan for optimal periodontal health and stability. It is also important to remember that occlusal stability cannot be obtained without muscle and joint stability. These two thoughts are clearly identified in Figure 8.16.

EXAMPLES OF COMPLEX CASES AND THEIR TREATMENT PLANNING PROCESS

Case 1—Perio-Prosthesis

This case (figs. 8.17–8.28) has survived over 20 years, even though the patient had suffered the ravages of periodontal disease and multiple missing teeth, broken down teeth, and multiple endodontically treated teeth. Because of the high risk associated with these potentially restored teeth, the basic occlusal scheme had to be planned out carefully and the finished result had to be extremely stable. The following items must be taken into consideration whenever treating this type of case:

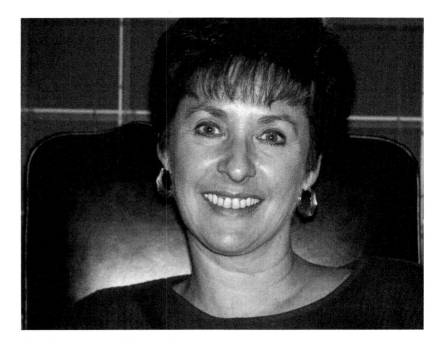

Fig. 8.17. Pre-op full face smiling view.

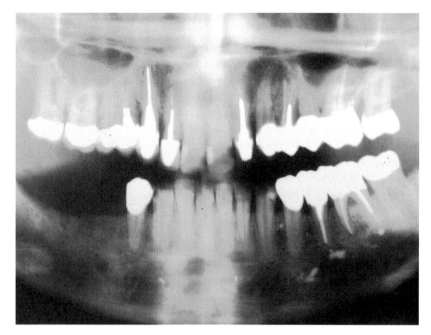

Fig. 8.18. Panoramic radiograph (note extensive numbers of endodontically treated anterior teeth leading to increased risk).

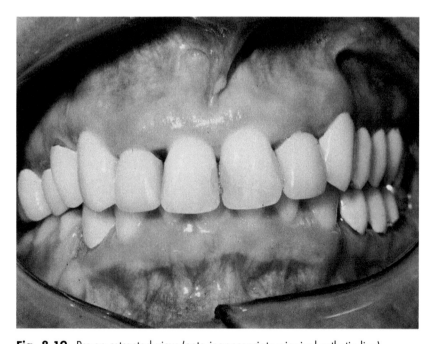

Fig. 8.19. Pre-op retracted view (note inappropriate gingival esthetic line).

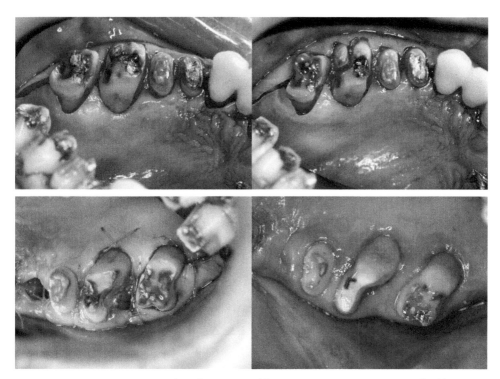

Fig. 8.20. Periodontal surgery addressing root amputation (note healthy tissue response around amputated molar).

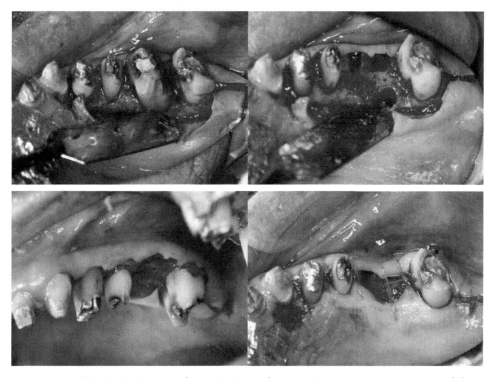

Fig. 8.21. Surgery demonstrating molar extraction as roots were poor candidates for amputations.

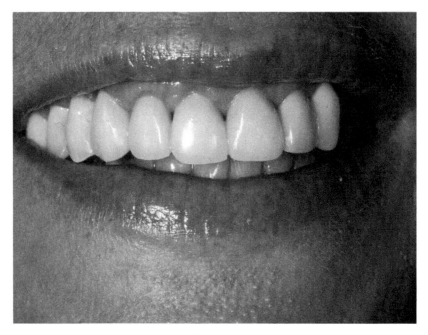

Fig. 8.22. Evaluating provisionals after crown lengthening.

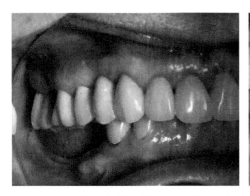
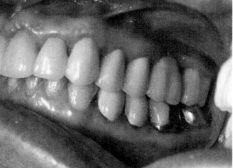

Fig. 8.23. Almost ready to take upper arch to completion—first need to reevaluate phonetics.

- Periodontal considerations
- Amount and quality of attached gingiva
- Amount of osseous support
- Type of osseous defects
- Mobility patterns/primary versus secondary
- Furcation involvement
- Root proximity problems
- Biologic width violations
- Ridge preservation/site development

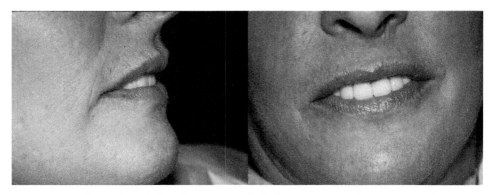

Fig. 8.24. Slight adjustment needed of maxillary incisal edges to produce easier phonetics (centrals need to roll over vermilion border).

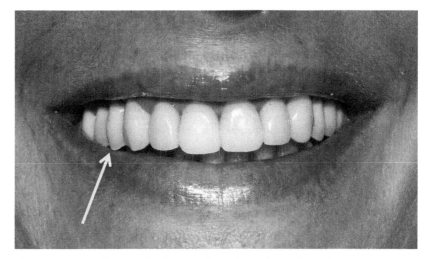

Fig. 8.25. Reevaluate smile plane and its relationship to lower lip.

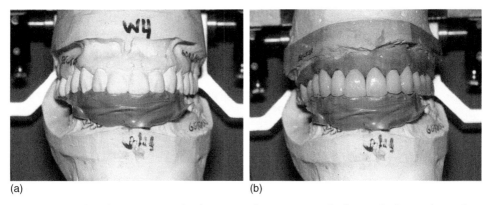

(a)   (b)

Fig. 8.26. a. Incisal edge matrix from provisionals. b. Finished porcelain edges matching incisal edge matrix. Note soft tissue model.

159

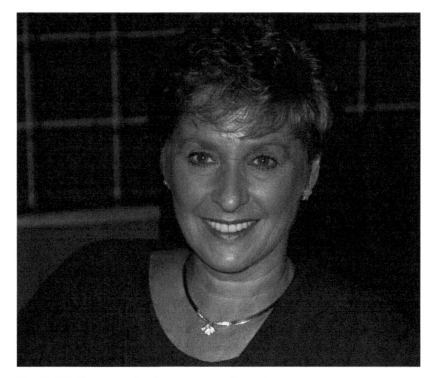

Fig. 8.27. Pleasant smile after two years of complex treatment.

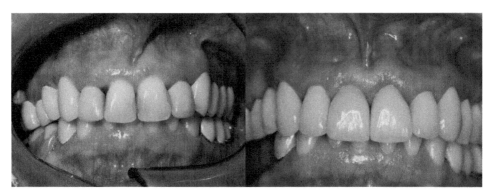

Fig. 8.28. Change in tissue contours, gingival height, and incisal edge position—all aided by esthetic plastic surgery.

Case 2—TMD, Wear, Pain, and Advanced Periodontal Issues Complicated by Esthetic Demands

This case has survived many years because of the stability achieved with the occlusal plane, centric stops, and strict hygiene maintenance, even though definitive periodontal surgery could not be accomplished except in one quadrant. However, the maintenance was a terrible problem for the patient and hygienists because of the residual deep pockets. Also note the excellent posterior disclusion of the molars but a compromised group function, due to the weakened condition of the maxillary cuspids. This type of case needs to have the following items taken into consideration:

- TMD (temporomandibular joint disorder) considerations
- Muscular versus intracapsular
- Emotional factors
- Bruxism/clenching
- Occlusal versus central nervous system
- Systemic arthritides
- Occlusal bite splint therapy

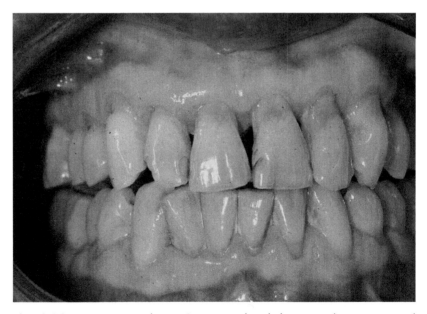

Fig. 8.29. Pre-op retracted view (note periodontal disease, esthetic issues, and functional problem).

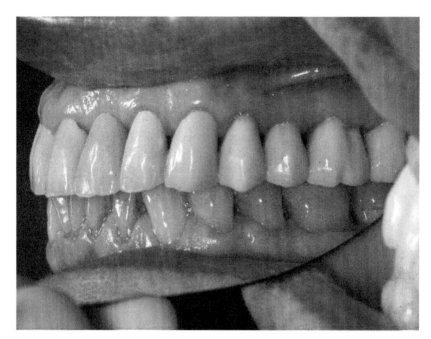

Fig. 8.30. Evaluating maxillary provisionals. (Patient has changed entire attitude and outlook with the provisionals. Chief concern has been answered.)

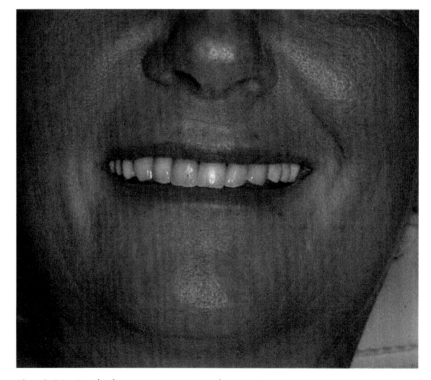

Fig. 8.31. Finished anterior ceramometal restorations.

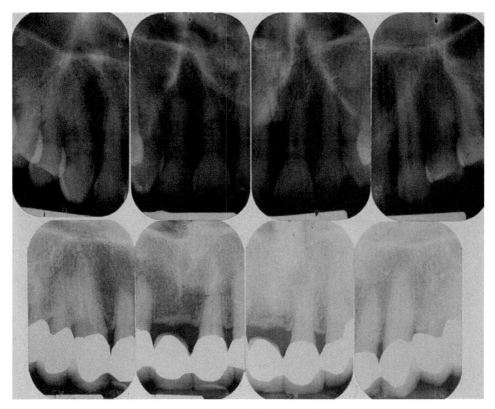

Fig. 8.32. Comparison of pre- and post-op radiographs.

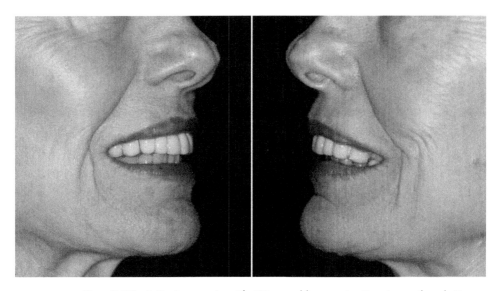

Fig. 8.33. Patient presents with 30-year-old reconstruction (even though it was falling apart, she loved its appearance).

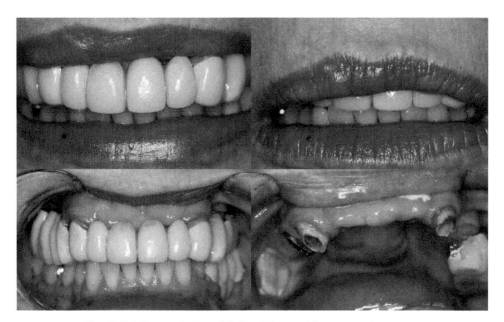

Fig. 8.34. Intraoral view of failing 30-year-old reconstruction.

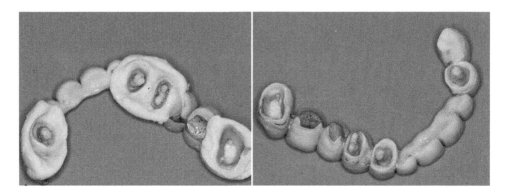

Fig. 8.35. Use of the failed reconstruction as the interim provisional is relined and trimmed.

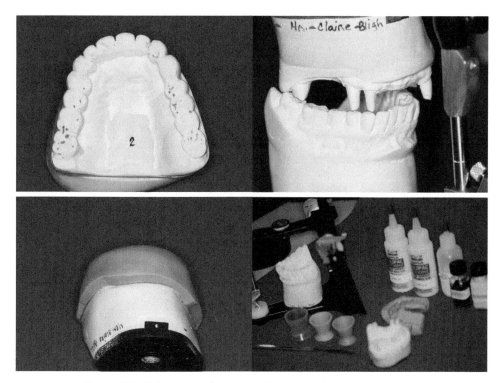

Fig. 8.36. Fabrication of custom cold cure acrylic provisionals.

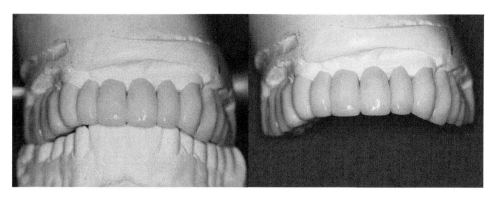

Fig. 8.37. Custom provisionals based on diagnostic workup.

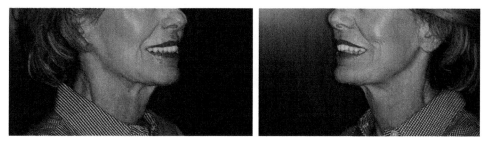

Fig. 8.38. Patient approval of provisionals.

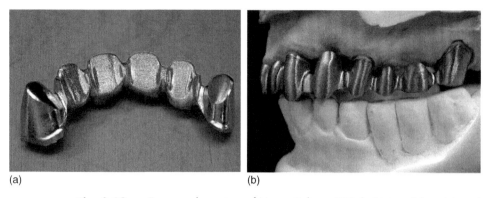

(a)   (b)

Fig. 8.39. a. Framework courtesy of Manny Palgon, CDT. b. Note solid model used for assembly, contours, emergence profile, and occlusion verification.

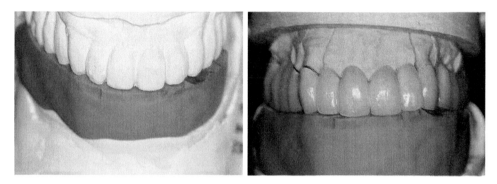

Fig. 8.40. Incisal edge matrix from provisionals to guide ceramist in creating precise anterior edge position and thickness.

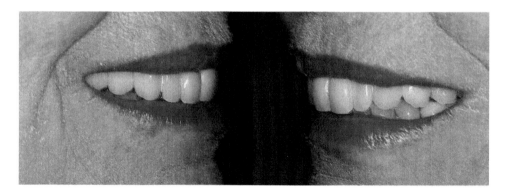

Fig. 8.41. Finished ceramometal reconstruction holding up for over 20 years.

REFERENCES

Amsterdam, M. (1974). Periodontal prosthesis: Twenty-five years in retrospect. *Alpha Omega*, Vol. 67, pp. 8–52.

Dawson, P.E. (1973). Temporomandibular joint pain–dysfunction problems can be solved. *Journal of Prosthetic Dentistry*, Vol. 29, pp. 100–112.

Dawson, P.E. (1999). Position paper regarding diagnosis, management, and treatment of temporomandibular disorders. *Journal of Prosthetic Dentistry*, Vol. 81, pp. 174–178.

Kirveskarari, P., Alanen, P., and Jamsa, T. (1989). Association between craniomandibular disorders and occlusal interferences. *Journal of Prosthetic Dentistry*, Vol. 62, pp. 66–69.

Mann, A.W., and Pankey, L.D. (1960) Oral rehabilitation. *Journal of Prosthetic Dentistry*, Vol. 10, pp. 135–162.

Schuyler, C.H. (1961). Factors contributing to traumatic occlusion. *Journal of Prosthetic Dentistry*, Vol. 11, pp. 708–715.

Schuyler, C.H. (2001). The function and importance of incisal edge guidance in oral rehabilitation. *Journal of Prosthetic Dentistry*, Vol. 86, pp. 219–232.

Spear, F.M. (2002). Occlusion in the new millennium: The controversy continues. *Signature*, Vol. 7, pp. 18–21.

Occlusal Bite Splint Therapy

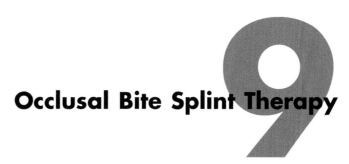

Roger A. Solow, DDS

The Glossary of Prosthodontic Terms (Academy of Prosthodontics, 2005) defines *occlusal device* as "any removable artificial occlusal surface used for diagnosis or therapy affecting the relationship of the mandible to the maxillae." The author uses the term *occlusal bite splint* (OBS) because it is more specific.

The OBS covers and gives the dentist control of the occlusal surface while connecting the supporting teeth. There are a variety of other terms—nightguard, orthotic, bite appliance, and splint—that have the same meaning without indicating a specific design.

PHILOSOPHY OF PATIENT CARE WITH OCCLUSAL BITE SPLINT THERAPY

Optimal dentistry can be defined as the education, diagnosis, and treatment that restores the patient to the highest level of comfort, function, and esthetics over the long term, with minimal maintenance. Attaining the best result requires that every aspect of care be performed with consistent excellence and attention to detail. The time invested to develop a relationship and understand the patient during the preclinical interview is the first step toward appropriate treatment. Clinical examination, occlusal analysis of diagnostic casts verified in centric relation (CR), and appropriate imaging are then done to define a problems list prior to treatment.

Comprehensive Occlusal Concepts in Clinical Practice, by Irwin M. Becker
© 2011 Blackwell Publishing Ltd.

Every dentist has an underlying philosophy that determines how each of these steps is performed. The amount of time spent with the patient, the type of technique, and the knowledge level of the dentist all relate to this philosophy. Many dentists have not thought about why they have a particular style of practice and are not aware of a more predictable and productive way to provide a higher quality of dentistry.

Comprehensive care is the codiagnosis and treatment of all factors that cause breakdown and loss of structure from bacterial challenge or excessive physical force. Ethical dentistry starts by giving patients a thorough description of their oral status, showing each area of health or disease. It is essential that patients completely understand their problems if they are to make informed decisions about definitive treatment. Patients will not commit extensive time, energy, or money unless they can visualize the final result and appreciate the implications of delaying treatment. OBS therapy has the primary role in educating patients about their occlusal problems while protecting teeth, restoring comfortable muscle coordination, and verifying the diagnosis.

Patients must be involved in their dental care to attain an optimal result. Procedures have limited significance unless the patient learns something. Codiagnosis, or patient education, is a conversation where each aspect of health or disease is shown and discussed. For example, prevention is the top priority in dentistry, as there is no value to restoring teeth unless the cause of breakdown is controlled. Teaching patients about home care is most effective when they are shown in their own mouth what plaque is and what it does, they perform the technique, and then any details are corrected. Clinical charting, diagnostic casts, full mouth x-rays, and photographs are discussed in the same detailed manner to educate and involve the patient.

OBS therapy follows this philosophy of care. Prior to treatment, diagnostic casts that are exact anatomic replicas of the mouth are reviewed, so that the occlusal problems are visualized. The dentist is responsible for identifying a specific diagnosis before recommending or performing treatment.

As a preview, an example of a meticulously refined OBS can be compared with an inadequate one. At delivery, time is taken to perfect the occlusion for a comfortable and predictable result. The patient is asked to describe how the bite feels with and without the OBS. Criticism and patient feedback are solicited. Postoperative appointments are scheduled until all details are corrected and an optimum result is achieved. The time dedicated to details and the participation in their treatment create a new experience for patients and promote acceptance of definitive care.

OBS therapy is a conservative, reversible treatment that is done prior to more invasive definitive treatment, when possible. It is an integral component of comprehensive care. A significant advantage of OBS therapy is the learning experience it creates for both the dentist and patient. The patient can preview the proposed occlusal correction and can remove the OBS to immediately return to the pretreatment state. The patient does not have to commit to definitive or invasive treatment to achieve occlusal stability or comfort.

OBS therapy permits the dentist to verify the occlusal analysis and diagnosis. Does the proposed occlusion give the expected result? Are muscles more comfortable when the traumatic occlusal interferences are removed? Is the range of mandibular motion improved? Can the temporomandibular joints (TMJs) tolerate normal load? Are teeth less mobile or sensitive?

The astute clinician evaluates the patient response as well as the oral status at each stage of treatment. A positive response—resolution of pathological signs and symptoms with appreciation from the patient—gives the dentist confidence to proceed. Negative responses are a warning not to proceed.

Patients who don't comply with using the OBS, show no resolution of pain, express no appreciation for the dentist's effort to perfect the OBS, are not cooperative with keeping appointments or financial commitments, and/or express irrational effects of treatment are likely to have a similar negative response with a more invasive and expensive approach.

Knowing the patient is a prerequisite to recommending definitive treatment. Does the patient accept responsibility for his or her problem or is someone else at fault? Accepting responsibility and a positive response to the OBS qualifies the patient for further treatment.

The OBS should be durable and provide protection for the dentition for the long term. The OBS can last for more than ten years with no loss of stability and minimal adjustment or wear. Just as exquisite provisional restorations for fixed prosthodontics are much more than a piece of plastic, OBS therapy is a full-mouth occlusal rehabilitation in a removable modality. A thorough knowledge of dental occlusion, the TMJs, and masticatory muscle anatomy, biomechanics, and pathology is required for excellence with OBS therapy. A poorly done OBS, reflecting minimal time or skill, causes a new malocclusion that is contrary to the desired goal. Dental fees should be structured so the dentist has the time needed to produce a stable, comfortable OBS with a perfected occlusion.

GOALS OF OCCLUSAL BITE SPLINT THERAPY

The goals of OBS therapy are to protect teeth or restorations, redistribute the forces when teeth contact, and preview the patient response to definitive treatment. These occlusal forces can affect all parts of the stomatognathic system. Force levels that exceed the physiologic tolerance of the system are responsible for breakdown of the teeth, periodontium, masticatory muscles, and TMJs. OBS therapy is indicated for occlusal problems affecting all of these areas.

Occlusal trauma causes tooth wear, fracture, mobility, migration, and pain to normally tolerated pressure and temperature. Loss of cervical enamel and dentin has been attributed to excess tensile stress from occlusal contacts (Grippo, 1991; Lee and Eakle, 1984, 1996; Braem, Lambrechts, and Vanherle, 1982).

Periodontal bone loss adjacent to implants is directly related to shear stress from occlusal contact (Oh et al., 2002; Steigenga, et al., 2004). Occlusal trauma is a risk factor in crestal bone loss in the natural dentition (McGuire and Nunn, 1996; Nunn and Harrel, 2001a, 2001b; Harrel, 2006) as the periodontal ligament (PDL) does not have an infinite capacity to shield crestal bone from stress. Clenching habits can fatigue elevator muscles, resulting in pain and decreased range of motion. Efforts to avoid occlusal interferences cause painful masticatory muscle incoordination from the simultaneous activation of elevator and protrusive muscle groups (Dawson, 1973; Juniper, 1984). Bruxing forces absorbed by the TMJ disturb the synovial fluid lubrication, affect disc displacement, and then load soft retrodiscal tissues (Nitzan, 2001; Nitzan and Marmary, 1997; Stegenga, 2000). Condylar bony change has been correlated with self-reported parafunctional habits (Israel et al., 1999; Yamada et al., 2001).

Optimizing occlusal forces can improve clinical signs and symptoms throughout the stomatognathic system (Tarantola et al., 1998; Kerstein and Farrell, 1990; Kerstein and Wright, 1991; Solow, 2005). OBS therapy can preview an optimal occlusion that could be achieved with equilibration, restoration, orthodontics, or orthognathic surgery.

Historically it was taught that OBS therapy was required to record accurate maxillomandibular records in CR (Roth, 1973; Dyer, 1973; Johnston and EICO, 1988). This adds time and cost to initial diagnostic procedures. Diagnostic casts verified in CR facilitate the fabrication of the OBS in CR and minimize chair time at delivery. Hands-on instruction with bimanual guidance provides consistent accuracy with CR records (Tarantola, Becker, and Gremillion, 1997; McKee, 1997). The use of an anterior deprogrammer (mini-OBS) facilitates taking accurate, repeatable CR records (Lundeen, 1974; Becker et al., 1999; Solow, 1999; McKee, 2005). For this author, using the anterior deprogrammer with bimanual guidance to record CR is a predictable procedure. The criteria to verify that CR is achieved are a consistent arc of closure of the lower incisor against the anterior deprogrammer, with bimanual guidance or with the patient's own power, and complete comfort in the TMJs.

If these criteria cannot be met due to pain in the TMJ region or tense masticatory muscles creating a variable arc of closure, then the patient is not in CR. OBS therapy is then essential to eliminate occlusal interferences and allow muscle relaxation so that the condyle can fully seat in its physiologic position. At this point, the dentist will feel the same loose and relaxed mandibular motion when the patient closes in CR against the OBS or against the anterior deprogrammer.

It is essential that the OBS be retentive and stable. The OBS must have zero mobility or it will not be comfortable or possible to create a precise occlusal contact scheme during function. Whether the OBS is fabricated by a laboratory or by the dentist, the most practical way to ensure proper retention with zero mobility is to intraorally reline the OBS with acrylic resin. Retention is adjusted by contouring the acrylic resin contacting the lingual undercuts. Metal clasps are not needed.

The rationale for creating precise occlusal contact scheme on the OBS is to control adverse forces from the existing occlusion. The same anatomic and biomechanical basis for an optimum occlusion of the natural dentition applies to the OBS:

1. All teeth should simultaneously contact the OBS with even pressure on mandibular closure with the condyles in CR. Even force distribution on multiple teeth minimizes force on each tooth and avoids occlusal trauma to a single tooth that causes protective mandibular displacement with muscle hyperactivity. Once the condyles are seated in CR, the lateral pterygoid muscles can relax without having to brace the mandible in a forward position (Mahan et al., 1983; Gibbs et al., 1984). The condyle seating in CR is a physiologic position in line with the vector of force of elevator muscles (Radu, Marandici, and Hottel, 2004). The condyles will achieve this position during power closure unless there is an occlusal interference, protrusive muscle splinting, or disc displacement. A consistent arc of closure is attained when both condyles are seated in CR. This shows as even-intensity dots on the OBS, consistently marking in the same position. (See figs. 9.1a and 9.1b.)

2. Posterior teeth and periodontium should be exposed to only vertical force and not contact the OBS in any jaw excursion to avoid traumatic lateral torque. The majority of periodontal membrane fibers have an oblique orientation and are designed to take vertical force (Grant, Stern, and Everett, 1972). The mandible functions as a Class III lever

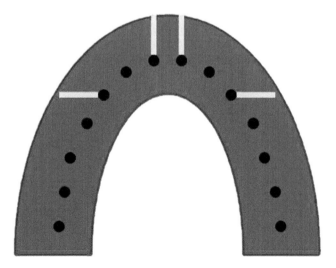

Fig. 9.1a. Maxillary occlusal bite splint (OBS) occlusal contact scheme.

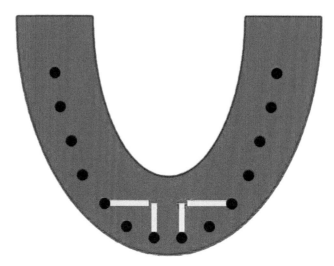

Fig. 9.1b. Mandibular OBS occlusal contact scheme (black dots = CR contacts; yellow lines = excursive contacts).

system with heavier forces on the posterior teeth than the anterior teeth. Excursive contact on posterior teeth creates significant torque that is transferred to the periodontium. Optimal force distribution avoids this type of contact. This shows as an absence of lines adjacent to posterior tooth dots on the OBS.

3. Anterior teeth should contact the OBS smoothly in all jaw excursions to slightly separate the posterior teeth. Anterior root inclination is less vertical than posterior root inclination, so only anterior teeth should contact in excursions for optimal stress distribution. Anterior crowns are in line with the root and have smooth surfaces that are designed for a gliding contact. In a Class III lever system there is less force farther away from the fulcrum (TMJ), so anterior teeth should contact in excursions for favorable stress distribution. This shows on the OBS as smooth, continuous lines adjacent to the dots of the anterior teeth to the full extent of border movement.

OCCLUSAL BITE SPLINT DESIGN

Hard methylmethacrylate resin is recommended to fabricate the OBS because it is a stable material, easy to reline or resurface, has proper retention, and can be refined to a precise occlusion. Soft OBSs are mobile, cannot be refined to a precise occlusion, and increase temporalis and masseter muscle activity (figs. 9.2 and 9.3; Okeson, 1987; Al Quran and Lyons, 1999).

Posterior tooth displacement from maxillary sinus problems is an indication for a soft vinyl OBS (Dawson, 1989). A hard OBS to retain the original tooth position could also be used in these cases to prevent displacement

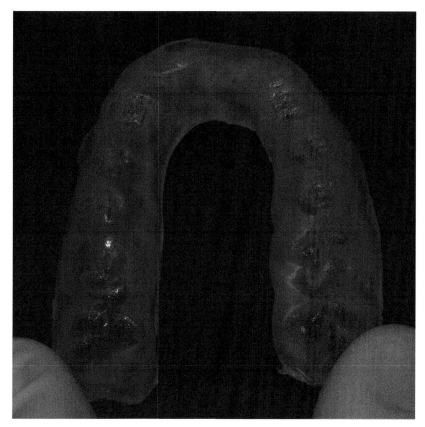

Fig. 9.2. Maxillary soft OBS (Note worn facet areas in all posterior teeth contact sites and rough border.).

after the teeth are repositioned. Either clear or light color acrylic resin can be used. Clear acrylic resin is less noticeable and allows direct visual confirmation of complete seating as the OBS clicks into place. Light color acrylic resin develops less stain from food and chromogenic bacteria over the long term.

OBSs can be made to fit on the maxillary or mandibular arch. The same technique and principles of design are used for both. The OBS should cover the arch with the most missing teeth, uneven incisal plane, mobile teeth, or restorations that need protection. This is a practical way to maximize the number of occlusal contacts, support the weakest teeth, and develop the simplest and smoothest anterior guidance.

Patients may have a preference for a maxillary or mandibular OBS if they have been comfortable with a previous one. There are advantages to both the maxillary and mandibular OBS. The maxillary OBS may be preferred in patients with lingually inclined posterior teeth where the flanges of the mandibular OBS restrict space for the tongue. For patients with a

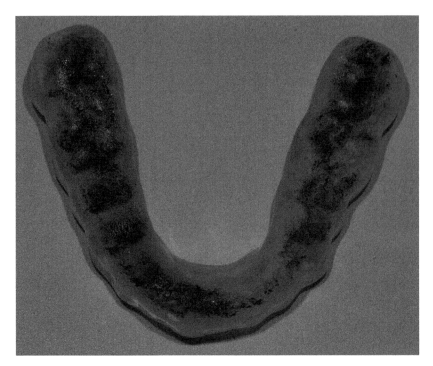

Fig. 9.3. Mandibular soft OBS (Note varying intensity of articulating ribbon marks over large areas of posterior teeth contact sites.).

retrognathic lower jaw and anterior open bite, the maxillary OBS has the anterior teeth centric stops and flat plane for anterior guidance located palatally compared to a mandibular design, which can extend more labially and distend the lip. Alternatively, a mandibular OBS with progressive contact in excursions starting on the canines followed by the incisors in protrusion or lateral protrusion can be made for these patients.

Mandibular OBSs are smaller and can be easier for some patients to tolerate. Patients who cannot comfortably close their lips around the properly contoured anterior aspect of a maxillary OBS may prefer a lower design. In patients with a prognathic lower jaw, a mandibular OBS will contact the maxillary anterior teeth with minimal facial acrylic resin extending toward the lip.

OBS design can be categorized as permissive or directive (Dawson, 1989). Permissive design allows the mandible a full range of motion in all directions, while a directive design restricts this range of motion. An anterior repositioning splint that protrudes the mandible with a steep anterior ramp to prevent the condyles from seating in CR is a directive design. A flat plane OBS, with even posterior teeth contact and anterior guidance that separates posterior teeth in all excursions to the full extent of border movement is a permissive design.

The OBS can cover an entire dental arch or a segment of the arch. Since human teeth erupt continually unless opposed by an equal force, full arch coverage is required. Segmental coverage allows a simultaneous intrusion of teeth by elevator muscle force through the covered teeth and extrusion of teeth not covered. This can permanently alter the plane of occlusion and require extensive restoration, segmental osteotomy, or orthodontic correction. Segmental coverage concentrates force on fewer teeth during bruxism episodes, resulting in higher forces, mobility, and discomfort on these teeth.

Separating posterior teeth with only anterior teeth coverage increases the force through the TMJs since no posterior teeth absorb force on closure (Ito et al., 1986). This may not be comfortable or appropriate for TMJs that are injured or have displaced discs with innervated retrodiscal tissues subject to load. Coverage of only anterior teeth can intrude the upper and lower anteriors to the thickness of the plastic layer and let the posterior teeth erupt. This results in an uneven or two-step occlusal plane on removal of the appliance. Orthodontists use this design to their advantage when the patients present with problems that would benefit from posterior tooth eruption and anterior tooth intrusion. A modified Hawley retainer with palatal acrylic resin contacting the only the lower anterior teeth is a common example (figs. 9.4 and 9.5; Rehany and Stern, 1981).

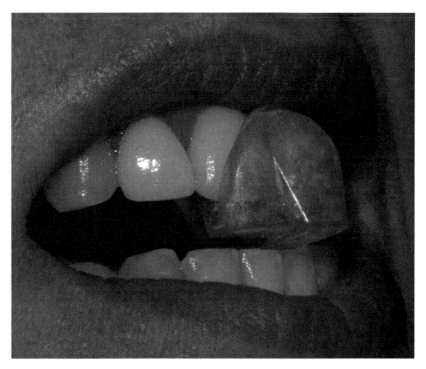

Fig. 9.4. Anterior segmental OBS (Note dimension of posterior open occlusal relation.).

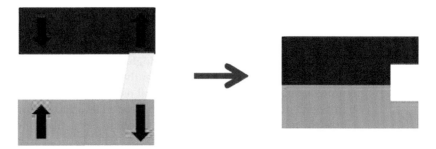

Fig. 9.5. Diagram of the possible effect of anterior segmental OBS use creating an anterior open occlusal relation (yellow = acrylic resin OBS; black arrows = forces on teeth and alveolar bone; blue = maxillary and mandibular dental arches).

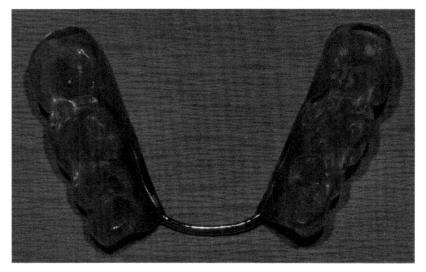

Fig. 9.6. Posterior segmental OBS (Note facets of wear and indents of maxillary buccal and lingual cusps.).

Separating anterior teeth with only posterior teeth coverage places all lateral excursion stress on posterior teeth, which is an unfavorable force distribution. The anterior teeth can then overerupt and are displaced lingually by the muscular lip force, while the posterior teeth are intruded to the thickness of the plastic coverage (figs. 9.6 and 9.7). Simply removing the segmental appliance will not allow the teeth to reerupt into their former position, and orthodontics is required to correct this malocclusion.

Segmental coverage might be given with the instruction to wear it only at night to avoid the risk of occlusal plane change. If patients do not follow instructions, significant occlusal problems can occur. Only full-arch OBSs

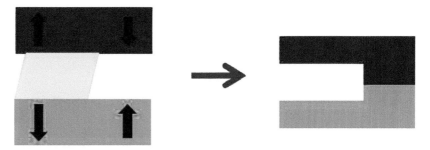

Fig. 9.7. Diagram of the possible effect of posterior segmental OBS creating a posterior open occlusal relation (yellow = acrylic resin OBS; black arrows = forces on teeth and alveolar bone; blue = maxillary and mandibular dental arches).

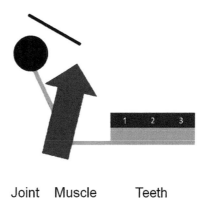

Joint   Muscle   Teeth

Fig. 9.8. Diagram of mechanical relation of the jaws as a Class III lever system (Whether the teeth contact at site 1 [molars], site 2 [premolars], or site 3 [anterior teeth], the vector of elevator muscle force will always seat the mandibular condyle against the articular eminence. Blue = maxillary and mandibular dental arches; red arrow = muscle force; black circle = condyle; black line = articular eminence.).

are recommended to avoid occlusal plane changes and pain in teeth, masticatory muscles, or the TMJs.

The pivot appliance is a segmental design that was touted to distract the condyle away from the mandibular fossa to alleviate pain from pressure on innervated soft tissue (Sears, 1956; Lous, 1978). A single molar contact on each side was supposed to cause a rotation on mandibular closure that would distract the condyle. The mandible functions as a Class III lever with the TMJ as the fulcrum, the muscle component anterior to the TMJ, and the teeth anterior to muscle (fig. 9.8). Since the muscle component is between the TMJ and teeth, when teeth do contact, any further contraction of the muscle will seat the condyle. External force anterior to the pivot area, in a superior direction, is required to distract the condyle inferior to the mandibular fossa.

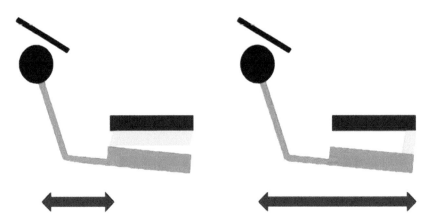

Fig. 9.9. Diagram of the shortened resistance lever arm from a molar OBS that reduces force to the TMJ compared to an incisor OBS (blue = maxillary and mandibular dental arches; black = TMJ; yellow = acrylic resin OBS; red = length of resistance lever arm.).

This is true no matter where the tooth contact is—molar, premolar, or incisor area. Physics dictate that there is no way to distract the condyle with only elevator muscle contraction. Pain relief may have been due to more even contact on the molars than the occlusal interferences in the dentition or reduced TMJ intraarticular pressure. Nitzan (1994) demonstrated that a uniform-thickness maxillary OBS with only molar contact reduced the resistance lever arm to the TMJ fulcrum and decreased TMJ intraarticular pressure by 81% (fig. 9.9).

A variety of segmental coverage designs have been suggested as a solution for temporomandibular disorders (TMDs) instead of full-arch OBS therapy. Segmental coverage has the disadvantages of intruding the teeth that support it, extruding the teeth it does not contact, increased pressure in the TMJ from lack of posterior teeth contact and an increased length of the resistance arm, heavy torque pressure on opposing posterior teeth when anterior teeth do not contact, or being swallowed. Only full-coverage design for the OBS is recommended.

The thickness of the OBS is a balance between fracture resistance and comfort to the lips and tongue. The molar acrylic resin should be 1–2 mm thick to prevent fracture. The anterior thickness will be greater since the jaw closes in an arc. Patients will not comply with an OBS that disturbs comfortable lip closure. Variations in anterior guidance design can minimize the problem of lip closure over the OBS (figs. 9.10a, 9.10b, and 9.10c).

There are a variety of OBS designs. It is essential that all of the above goals and principles of optimum design are incorporated in OBS therapy to avoid adverse effects in the stomatognathic system. A two-splint design, the dual B (bruxism) splint, is a flat appliance on one arch opposed by a

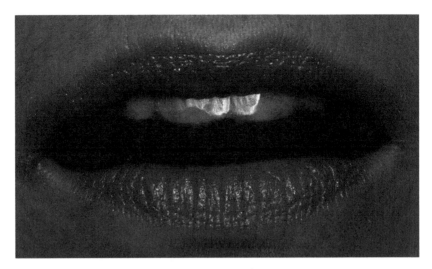

Fig. 9.10a. Thick maxillary OBS to maximize fracture resistance.

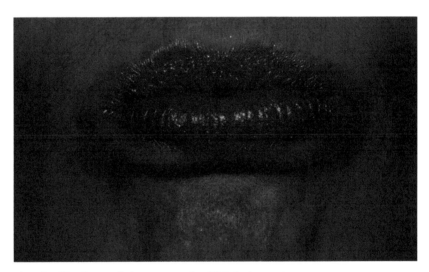

Fig. 9.10b. Strained closure over the OBS thick anterior contour.

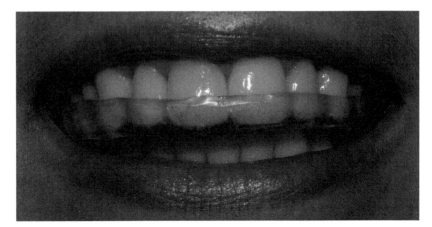

Fig. 9.10c. Significant reduction of the entire occlusal surface thickness allowing comfortable lip closure and compliance with nightly use.

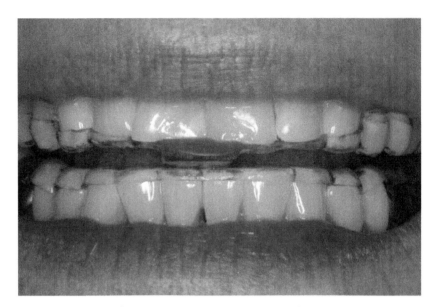

Fig. 9.11. Dual B (bruxism) OBS (Note both dental arches are covered to avoid intrusion-/extrusion-related occlusal plane problems. Only the maxillary anterior ramp is adjusted.).

flat appliance with a ramp on the incisors of the opposing arch (fig. 9.11). This design uses the same principle as intraoral pantographic clutches to disengage the teeth, allow a permissive contact in all excursions between the incisor ramp and the opposing plastic, and permit the condyles access to CR. It has the advantage of adjusting only one area of occlusal contact but requires both arches to be covered (Wilkerson, 2009).

OCCLUSAL BITE SPLINT FABRICATION

The recommended procedure for OBS fabrication follows:

1. Duplicate the diagnostic casts so the original casts are preserved in the patient record. Polyvinylsiloxane impression materials permit multiple accurate pours for duplicate casts. Irreversible hydrocolloid impressions can be used for accurate duplicate casts if they are kept moist during setting and are repoured within 45 minutes (Haywood and Powe, 1998). Mount the duplicate casts in CR with the same facebow, CR record, and protrusive record. The facebow transfers the radius of the patient's arc of closure to the diagnostic casts. After mounting, the casts can be verified in CR by placing the marked anterior deprogrammer on the casts and having the same point of closure of the lower incisor that was present intraorally and on the

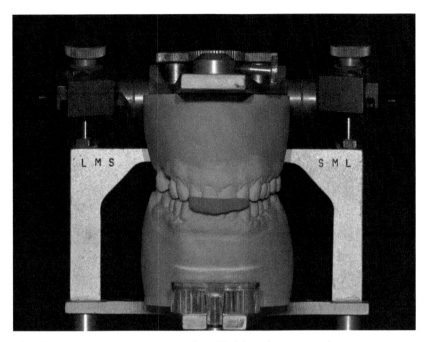

Fig. 9.12. Diagnostic casts mounted in CR (Note the anterior deprogrammer, initially formed intraorally, repositioned on the casts to verify that the lower incisor contact is identical to that during CR registration with bimanual guidance.).

original diagnostic casts (fig. 9.12; Solow, 1999). If these records are not available, use a wax transfer record.

2. Lute utility wax on the cast to form the borders of the OBS and contain the acrylic resin (fig. 9.13). Set the pin on the semiadjustable articulator to allow 1–2 mm thickness of material at the second molar. This dimension allows occlusal adjustment without a thin, fracture-prone area. Lubricate the cast liberally to allow for OBS removal without damage.

3. Mix methylmethacrylate resin until doughy and apply to the cast within the wax border. Close the articulator until the pin touches (fig. 9.14). Remove the cast and place, with the acrylic, into a pressure pot (fig. 9.15). Cure for ten minutes at 30 psi to decrease porosity.

4. Remove the OBS from the cast and mark the borders and centric contacts of the opposing teeth with a pencil. Trim off the excess acrylic on a lathe-mounted stone wheel and replace on the articulated cast. Refine the occlusion with an acrylic bur until there are uniform, even marks in CR on all teeth. Move the casts through all excursions and flatten any acrylic marking adjacent to the CR contact dots (figs. 9.16a and 9.16b). Refine the anterior teeth contact until smooth lines are evident from the canine and central incisor CR contacts out to the full

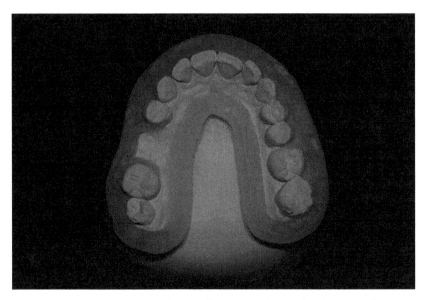

Fig. 9.13. Utility wax luted to the maxillary cast to form a border that will contain the acrylic resin during OBS fabrication (The facial position should allow one-third tooth coverage by the OBS for retention.).

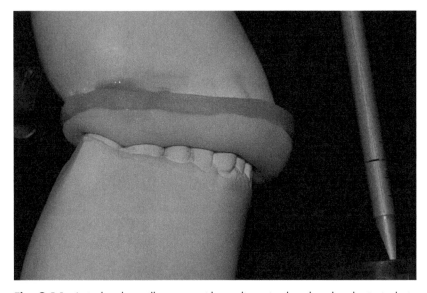

Fig. 9.14. Articulated maxillary cast with acrylic resin closed so that the incisal pin touches the platform (This ensures that the OBS will have predetermined proper thickness for fracture resistance.).

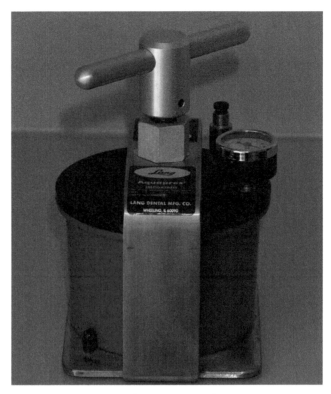

Fig. 9.15. Acrylic resin OBS cured under pressure for 10 minutes at 30 psi to reduce porosity (Aquapres, Lang Dental, Wheeling, IL).

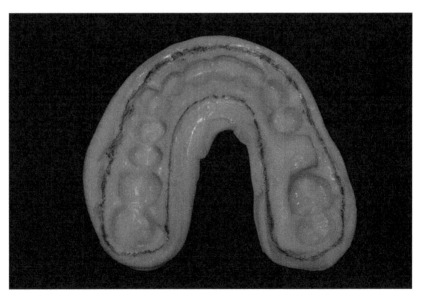

Fig. 9.16a. Intaglio surface of OBS after processing (Borders are marked for rapid contouring with lathe-mounted stone wheel.).

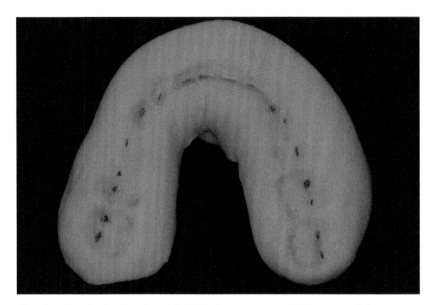

Fig. 9.16b. Occlusal surface of OBS after processing (CR contact of the anterior incisal edges and lower buccal cusps are marked. These marks are preserved during contouring.).

extent of border movement. It is a significant learning experience for dentists how ultra smooth anterior guidance can be created on the OBS while on the articulator (fig. 9.17).

5. Remove all septae and relieve the intaglio of the OBS to ensure complete seating and room for the acrylic resin reline. Alternatively, a thin wax layer can be placed prior to applying the acrylic on the cast.

6. Discuss with the patient that there will be a significant plastic taste for several minutes. Place a thin mix of the same acrylic used to fabricate the OBS in the relieved intaglio and seat with firm pressure on the teeth. Use an explorer to remove any excess acrylic resin beyond the facial border. Rinse the mouth with water to minimize the acrylic resin taste. Repetitively lift and seat the OBS, pulling on one molar border, to mold the acrylic so that it is shaped to rotate off on dislodgement (fig. 9.18). This creates resistance to vertical displacement and forms a retentive OBS that seats with a snap. Remove the OBS from the mouth prior to final set and let it bench cure for several minutes until completely hard (fig. 9.19).

7. Remove the interdental septae and excess reline acrylic past the borders of the OBS with an acrylic bur. Try in the OBS by orienting it over the anterior teeth and rotating it into place. Relieve any acrylic resin in undercut areas that prevent seating. The OBS must snap into place and have zero mobility. Relieve any acrylic resin area that feels too tight on a tooth.

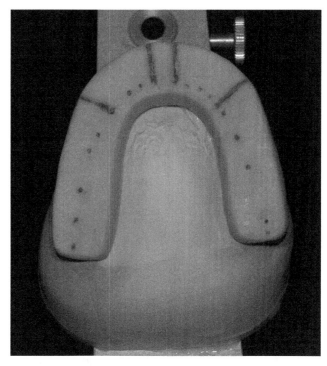

Fig. 9.17. Maxillary OBS on the articulator (The occlusion is refined with acrylic burs to achieve the occlusal scheme prior to intraoral reline. This allows chair time to be spent refining details instead of gross adjustment.).

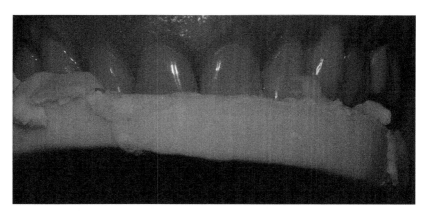

Fig. 9.18. Maxillary OBS rotated on and off one side during intraoral reline (This creates retention by resistance to vertical displacement and a snap-on full seating.).

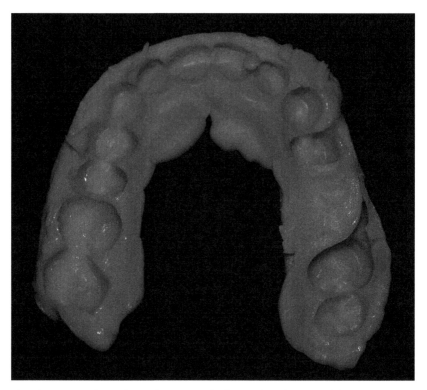

Fig. 9.19. Intaglio surface after intraoral reline with a thin mix of the same acrylic resin that was used to fabricate the OBS.

8. Place the patient in the supine position to facilitate the condyles closing in CR. Mark with red articulating ribbon as the patient closes on their own, without bimanual guidance, and adjust the OBS until all teeth contact (fig. 9.20a). Acrylic resin can be added to any site that is not contacting. After even contacts are marking on each tooth, use bimanual guidance to discern any premature contacts and adjust these until the patient cannot feel one side contact before the other. Even contacts show by equal intensity marks in each site. Use firm bimanual guidance without ribbon to close into the CR marks. Even contact will show by halos or clear centers in the existing marks and can be achieved literally within the thickness of an ink dot. This can be checked with 20u plastic articulating ribbon (fig. 9.20b) or 8u foil shimstock. Anterior teeth should contact slightly lighter than posterior teeth, as their roots are smaller. It is uncomfortable for the patient to contact heavier on anterior teeth than posterior teeth. Sit the patient upright and mark the anterior teeth as the patient closes on their own. There is a difference in condylar seating in the upright and supine positions. When the condyle is not fully seated with power closure in

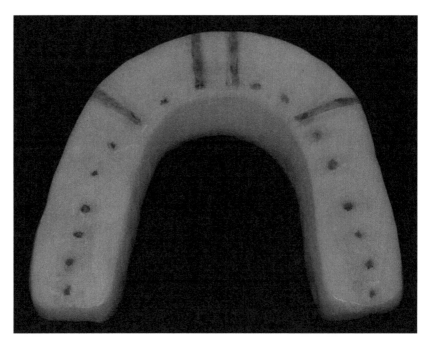

Fig. 9.20a. Maxillary OBS with occlusal contacts marked by silk ribbon (Madame Butterfly, Almore International, Beaverton, OR; red dots = CR contacts; blue lines = excursive contacts).

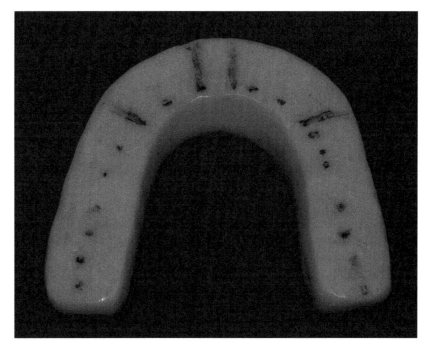

Fig. 9.20b. Same maxillary OBS with occlusal contacts marked by 20u mylar ribbon (Accufilm, Parkell, Farmingdale, NY).

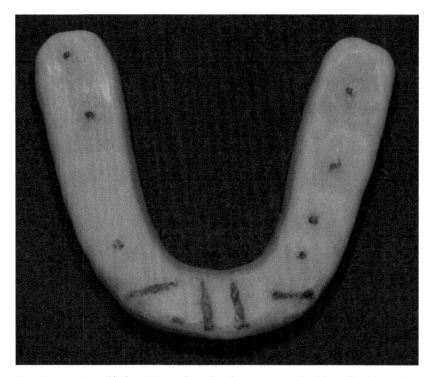

Fig. 9.20c. Mandibular OBS with occlusal contacts marked by silk ribbon (Red dots = CR contacts; blue lines = excursive contacts. Note lack of #29 and #30 contacts due to missing teeth #3 and #4.).

CR, the jaw will rotate in a slightly more anterior arc. Relieve any marks anterior to the CR contacts to provide a freedom of centric during closure. The acrylic resin immediately anterior to the CR marks should be flat and not inclined. This adjustment avoids the patient's feeling "locked in."

9. Place the patient in the supine position and mark with blue ribbon as the patient goes through all lateral, protrusive, and lateral protrusive excursions on their own without bimanual guidance (fig. 9.20c).

Remove any acrylic resin that marks lateral to any posterior tooth CR red dot. Smooth the anterior teeth blue marks so that continuous lines form adjacent to the red CR dots to the full extent of border movements. The dentist has control over which teeth take the force in excursions. A progressive contact of canines and then central incisors in lateral and protrusive excursion shares the stress on these teeth. If lower incisors have lost bone support or have minimal coronal dentin to support a crown, then the stronger canines should take all of the load in all excursions and the weak teeth should only have CR red dots. This maxillary OBS design has been termed the "Michigan

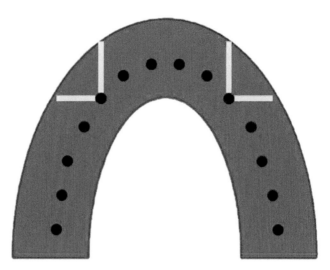

Fig. 9.21a. Diagram of maxillary occlusal contacts of the "Michigan Splint" design (Black dots = CR contacts; yellow lines = excursive contacts. Note absence of excursive contacts on the incisors.).

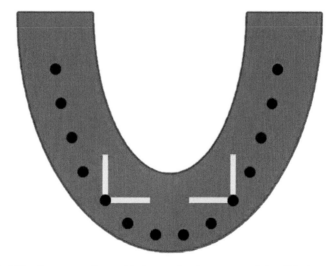

Fig. 9.21b. Diagram of mandibular occlusal contacts of the "Michigan Splint" design.

splint" (figs. 9.21a and 9.21b; Ramfjord and Ash, 1994). It has the advantages of simplifying the anterior guidance scheme with excursion lines adjacent to only the canines, minimizing anterior bulk of the OBS for comfort, and avoiding crowded lower anterior teeth for anterior guidance. It has the disadvantage of placing all force on the canines without sharing the force with the incisors. If a canine is compromised, then the stronger lateral and central incisors should contact in a group with incisal guidance to share the load with the canines (figs. 9.22a and 9.22b).

The mark from contact of the anterior contour of the OBS with the opposing teeth may appear as a dot, line, or area. All of these contacts

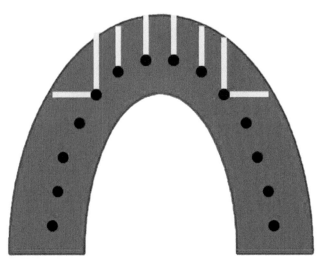

Fig. 9.22a. Diagram of maxillary OBS occlusal contacts with the anterior guidance shared by canines and incisors (black dots = CR contacts; yellow lines = excursive contacts).

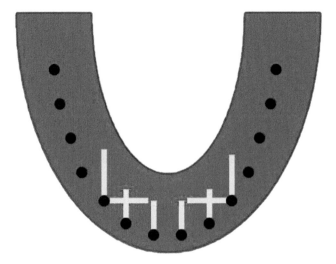

Fig. 9.22b. Diagram of the mandibular OBS with the anterior guidance shared by canines and incisors.

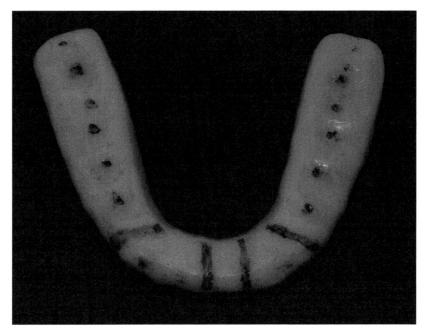

Fig. 9.23a. Mandibular OBS with a simplified occlusal scheme (black dots = CR contacts; blue lines = excursive contacts).

are acceptable as long as the anterior guidance is very smooth. If the posterior teeth have only CR contacts and the anterior teeth glide smoothly with no interrupting "catches" or "hitches," then the OBS has the optimum design. The dentist can then choose the anterior guidance scheme that distributes force on the appropriate teeth using the simplest design possible. For example, the mandibular OBS during lateral excursion past the canine contact into the crossover position may track along the straight protrusive mark with contact of the upper incisal edges, distal to mesial. The mark appears as a straight anterior-posterior line without a lateral direction like the canine (figs. 9.23a and 9.23b). Slight reduction of the acrylic resin adjacent to these marks creates a simplified anterior guidance occlusal scheme that is practical to achieve and provides ultra smooth anterior guidance in all directions.

Repeat all excursions under firm pressure with bimanual guidance on blue ribbon to detect contact that can occur with mandibular deformation similar to forceful bruxing (Okeson, Dickson, and Kemper, 1982).

10. Round the border of the OBS to avoid sharp edges. This curve will form smooth excursive contact to the full extent of border movement without extending the acrylic further toward the lip. This curve also

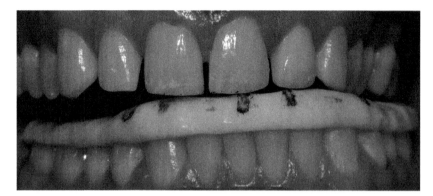

Fig. 9.23b. Mandibular OBS on left crossover excursion (Note the maxillary left central incisor contact in a smooth transition after the left canine finishes its excursive contact. The straight anterior-posterior track on the central incisors also functions as the lateral protrusive and crossover excursion contact with the maxillary central incisal edges.).

allows progressive contact of the central incisors as the opposing canines travel apically beyond the border of the OBS to the crossover position. Smooth any sharp incisal edges of opposing teeth that will cut grooves into the softer acrylic resin and interrupt smooth anterior guidance paths. This avoids the need for amalgam or composite inserts designed to resist wear (Bonfante, Ramos, and Bonfante, 2003).

11. Ask the patient, "Is there anything not 100% comfortable to your tongue or bite?" and "Is there any detail that I can do better?" Once all refinement is finished, have the patient take out the OBS and compare the feel of the natural dentition. Patients who are involved in the process of creating an excellent OBS occlusion typically ask the dentist to create the same comfortable occlusion with equilibration or restoration.

12. Postoperative visits are essential to account for change that occurs at the level of the PDL or the TMJ. Teeth with widened PDLs from occlusal trauma will shift position or rebound as that force is removed with even contact on the OBS. Decreased inflammation and edema in the TMJ may allow superior movement of the condyle, resulting in heavier occlusal contacts on that side of the OBS on mandibular closure. Refinement with a rubber wheel will restore even CR contacts that can be verified with 20u ribbon, 8u shimstock, and patient comment. Two short postoperative appointments should be part of the OBS service. The first appointment should be ideally scheduled within 24 hours. Additional time should be scheduled if the patient thinks the even contact of all teeth on closure or the smooth anterior guidance can be improved. The occlusion on the OBS is monitored at periodic cleaning and exam appointments.

13. Maintenance instructions should stress that anytime the OBS is not in the mouth it needs to be in a container. Loss of the OBS involves significant time, effort, and expense. Daily brushing of the OBS is recommended to minimize plaque and calculus formation. A towel in the sink can prevent fracture if the OBS slips during brushing. This author prefers to keep the OBS wet when it is not being used to avoid any possible warping on drying and use effervescent tablets that help clean any porosities in the acrylic resin.

THE CLINICAL RESEARCH BASIS FOR OCCLUSAL BITE SPLINT THERAPY

All studies have limitations and must be critically analyzed prior to accepting their conclusions as reliable evidence for clinical practice. The literature does not provide every answer for clinical decisions, so the dentist must know anatomy, pathophysiology, and biomechanics to understand the occlusal basis for optimal patient care. This is especially true when similar studies yield conflicting conclusions. This section is a sample of the extensive clinical literature on OBS therapy.

OCCLUSAL BITE SPLINT THERAPY AND THE TEETH

OBS therapy is frequently prescribed in the presence of worn, mobile, and fractured teeth or restorations to protect teeth and redistribute occlusal forces (Clark, 1984a; Lytle, 2001). These forces generated by destructive tooth contacts have to be absorbed by the teeth and periodontium, with progressive adverse effects on both of these structures. The OBS can only protect teeth when it is used by the patient. For some patients, nocturnal wear may be sufficient since there is no conscious control of oral habits or clenching and grinding activity at that time. Patients with uncontrolled oral habits, severe myofascial pain, or TMJ pain may benefit from continual use, 24 hours a day. Progressive discomfort, wear, mobility, or fracture of teeth despite consistent nocturnal OBS use is indicative of daytime occlusal force problems, and 24-hour use prior to definitive care is recommended.

Patients commonly present with an OBS prescribed for TMDs and bruxism. TMD is a nonspecific term that refers to pain in the TMJ area or masticatory muscles, limited range of mandibular motion, and TMJ sounds. Studies evaluating the effect of OBS therapy on TMDs have limited value if a specific diagnosis is not made for each patient with clinical examination, appropriate imaging, and occlusal analysis of diagnostic casts mounted in CR. Most studies do not photograph or verify an optimal occlusion produced by the OBS. Over 95% of OBSs that patients bring in to this author's practice have a poor occlusion that alters the existing malocclusion instead of providing an optimal occlusion.

OCCLUSAL BITE SPLINT THERAPY EFFECT ON MASTICATORY MUSCLE

OBS therapy is consistently shown to reduce pain in the masticatory muscles and restore the symmetry of their activity. Scopel, Costa, and Urias (2005) evaluated the anterior temporalis and masseter electromyographic (EMG) activity of normal and myogenous TMJ patients. At rest, 85% of subjects maintained jaw position by using the anterior temporalis more than the masseters. The myogenous pain patients had higher resting EMG activity of the anterior temporalis and masseter muscles and a higher asymmetry than the normals. OBS therapy reduced the activity index of these muscles with complete remission of pain.

Okeson, Kemper, and Moody (1982) found that wearing a maxillary OBS improved pain and interincisal distance in patients with craniomandibular disorders. There was no difference between acute and chronic group response.

Barker (2004) evaluated 60 patients after treatment with a mandibular OBS, equilibrated so that all teeth made equal contact in CR with canine disclusion in protrusive and lateral excursions. Forty-six percent of patients had previous unsuccessful splint therapy. Ninety-five percent of patients experienced significant pain relief. Fifty-eight percent of patients had improved mandibular range of motion.

Emshoff and Bertram (1998) used ultrasound to evaluate the anterior temporalis, anterior and deep masseter, anterior and posterior digastric, and sternocleidomastoid muscles. OBS therapy reduced, in the short term, local muscle thickness and asymmetry.

Beard and Clayton (1980) evaluated 482 pantographic tracings on 15 experimental subjects and 5 controls who used OBS adjusted to centric relation and immediate canine disclusion. OBS therapy reinstated muscle coordination. They recommended occlusal adjustment after OBS therapy to maintain muscle coordination and to prevent reinsertion of occlusal interferences and the return of protective reflexes.

Kurita, Ikeda, and Kurashina (2000) evaluated 6 patients with masticatory muscle pain after four weeks of OBS therapy. Patients with either high or low initial occlusal force on the OBS normalized to the level of healthy subjects.

Jimenez (1987) studied the EMG activity of the masseter and anterior and posterior temporalis muscles clenching on CR interferences and in maximum intercuspation, with and without an OBS. Clenching on CR interferences inhibited masseter muscle activity and reduced anterior and posterior temporalis muscle activity compared to clenching on the OBS. If there is a premature contact on closure, the jaw muscles must contribute to stabilization and reduce the maximum contraction to avoid damage to structures involved in compensatory stabilization.

Humsi et al. (1989) evaluated 36 patients with a myogenous craniomandibular disorder after treatment with a maxillary OBS for day and night wear. Canine guidance in lateral excursions and anterior teeth guidance in protrusive excursions were provided. Properly adjusted OBSs immediately improved symmetry of masseter muscle activity. OBSs with minor occlusal interferences at the first recall showed decreased muscle symmetry from the time of delivery.

MASTICATORY MUSCLE ACTIVITY AND OBS GUIDANCE CONTACTS

Williamson and Lundquist (1983) measured temporalis and masseter muscle EMG activity during dynamic lateral excursions on an OBS with canine guidance or group function contact. Elevator muscle activity was reduced when the posterior teeth were discluded by canine guidance.

Shupe et al. (1984) showed that dynamic group function contact on the OBS produced 38% higher EMG activity of the elevator muscles compared to canine guidance contact. They recommended canine protected guidance during restoration to reduce forces on posterior teeth.

Fitins and Sheikholeslam (1993) found EMG activity of elevator muscles decreased significantly when biting on the canine ramp of the OBS compared to clenching in maximum intercuspation on the teeth or OBS.

Ramfjord and Ash (1994) recommended the OBS have canine guidance only, in all excursions to reduce elevator muscle activity.

Manns, Chan, and Miralles (1987) found that static and dynamic clenching on an OBS with canine guidance reduced elevator muscle compared to group function contact. They concluded that canine guidance has pressure concentrated in a small periodontal surface area, allowing less elevator muscle activity. They recommended canine guidance for OBS therapy. However, Graham and Rugh (1988) compared OBSs with canine or molar guidance and found the same EMG activity reduction during lateral excursions. They suggested there may be a mechanical benefit to using canine guidance clinically.

Rugh et al. (1989) tested the effect of canine versus molar guidance OBS therapy on 8 patients with a history of bruxism. Nocturnal masseter muscle EMG activity, clinical examination, and pain rating did not differ with the two guidance patterns.

OCCLUSAL BITE SPLINT THERAPY EFFECT ON THE TMJ

Clark (1984b) reviewed the literature for the effect of flat plane OBS on TMJ clicking, pain, and osteoarthritis. TMJ clicking was the most resistant symptom to treatment, and Clark questioned the need to correct clicking alone, if it is not progressive. Some relief of TMJ pain was noted, but the studies were few in number and inconsistent in results. The few clinical reports, without control patients, that suggest reversal of degenerative joint change, used repositioning splints. The need to remodel condyles simply because they are not ideal in form was questioned.

Tsuga et al. (1989) evaluated the effect of thirteen weeks of OBS therapy on 30 TMJ dysfunction patients. Eighty-seven percent of these patients reported improvement to pain on opening or chewing, 78% had reduction of TMJ sounds, 68% had improvement in the limitation of movement, and 86% had improved shoulder pain.

Carraro and Caffesse (1978) evaluated 170 patients for the response of symptoms with OBS therapy. Eighty percent had improved pain to palpation of the masticatory muscles and TMJ. Seventy-one percent had improved clicking, limited opening, and jaw incoordination.

WHY DOES OCCLUSAL BITE SPLINT THERAPY WORK?

Clark (1984a) and Dao and Lavigne (1998) reviewed the theories of why OBS therapy works: restored vertical dimension, maxillomandibular realignment, TMJ repositioning, cognitive awareness, and occlusal disengagement (providing an ideal occlusal scheme). They noted that there is no conclusive testing or acceptance of these theories.

Loss of vertical dimension can occur in partial and fully edentulous patients, especially with attrition of artificial teeth. In the natural dentition, compensatory eruption of teeth maintains vertical dimension to the repetitive contraction length of the elevator muscles. Hellsing (1984) evaluated ten patients with maxillary OBS and concluded that jaw muscle motor behavior is dynamic and adaptable to extreme changes in vertical dimension. Rapid adjustment of postural position is due to periodontal receptors and muscle spindles.

Carlsson, Ingervall, and Kocak (1979) cemented clear acrylic splints to the canines and posterior teeth of six subjects with no symptoms of TMD. Occlusion was refined to create stability in CR and smooth excursions with an increased vertical dimension of 3.9 mm. Immediately after placement of the splints, a new interocclusal distance was established. They concluded that postural position of the mandible varies according to conditions and is not acceptable as a basis for determining the occlusal vertical dimension.

Rugh and Drago (1981) studied 10 subjects free of masticatory muscle disease and found that, as vertical dimension increased, muscle activity decreased until a point of minimal activity and then increased. The minimal EMG activity at an average of 8.6 mm did not correlate with clinical rest position. They showed that jaw muscles were in slight contraction to maintain clinical rest position.

Manns et al. (1983) evaluated 75 patients with OBSs of 1 mm, 4.42 mm, and 8.15 mm intercisal distance. They found that splints near the vertical dimension of less EMG activity are more effective in promoting neuromuscular relaxation.

Loss of vertical dimension from mandibular overclosure is not a basis for OBS therapy. Compensatory eruption occurs in the worn dentition to maintain original vertical dimension. Vertical dimension is a variable position that is difficult to accurately assess clinically, and treatment at varying interincisal distances is therapeutic.

Maxillomandibular realignment refers to achieving a neuromuscular balance via bimanual guidance into CR, using cast landmarks of teeth and gingiva to create a proper OBS-determined position of the mandible, or using a muscle-determined approach with transcutaneous electrical nerve stimulation.

Schwartz, Kudyba, and Martine (1986) stated that the maxillary and mandibular midlines should approximate each other during hinge axis rotation if there are no points of restraint within the occlusal tables.

Fu et al. (2003) evaluated the effect of flat plane OBS therapy and alignment of the maxillary and mandibular labial frena on 20 adults, with and without TMDs. After OBS therapy, all patients had the mandibular position shift toward aligned maxillary and mandibular frena. Improved symmetry of the maxilla relative to the mandible with OBS therapy would be expected as occlusal interferences are removed and both condyles are allowed to seat without displacement in their fossae during elevator muscle contraction. However, skeletal asymmetry of the jaws, midline deviation from missing teeth, and TMJ asymmetry make cast landmarks an unreliable guideline.

TENS stimulation to establish the maxillomandibular relation was shown to create a variable mandibular position, inferior and anterior to CR, with an increased dimension of the rest position (Strohaver, 1972; Lundeen, 1974; Remien and Ash, 1974; Noble, 1975; Wessberg, Epker, and Elliott, 1983; Widmer, Lund, and Feine, 1990). The ideal maxillomandibular relation is CR since it allows for proper anatomic position of the mandibular condyle with the meniscus and articular eminence, as well as relaxation of the lateral pterygoid muscle. Bimanual guidance to record CR in the healthy TMJ is predictable and practical to achieve because it is based on the optimal functional anatomic relationship of the TMJ components and associated musculature (Dawson, 1985; McNeill, 1985). The occlusal goal of OBS therapy is even contact with all the teeth in CR, confirmed with bimanual guidance, restoring coordination with the components of the stomatognathic system.

TMJ repositioning is altering the position of the condyle in the fossa to improve TMJ function. Mongini (1980) demonstrated condylar remodeling after occlusal therapy with splints, equilibration, restoration, or orthodontics. Flattened condyles became rounded in 7 out of 11 patients, and degenerative arthritic changes in 3 patients became normal. There was no change in initially round condyles. Mongini concluded that occlusal alteration directly influences bony contours of the condyle and its position in the TMJ. This agrees with his earlier study of 100 skulls (Mongini, 1972), which showed that remodeling of the mandibular condyle is an adaptation of the bone structure to mechanical stresses derived from functional activity.

Williamson et al. (1977) found that flat plane OBS correction of the occlusion repositioned the condyles 1.0 mm anterior-superior in the normal group and 1.5 mm posterior-superior in the TMJ symptomatic group.

Israel et al. (1999) arthroscopically examined 124 TMJs in patients with witnessed or self-reported parafunction. Sixty-six percent of the joints had osteoarthritis from parafunction. They recommended that parafunctional activity be addressed nonsurgically to avoid abnormal joint loading that leads to osteoarthritis.

Wang et al. (2008) used a cadaver study to show that the TMJ disc alters its morphology in response to changes in condyle-fossa space caused by abnormal occlusion. They concluded that occlusal problems should be addressed in TMD patients with disc deformation.

These studies show that condylar position is directly related to the occlusion and that excess occlusal force has a destructive effect on the TMJ, which attempts to compensate by altering its form. Occlusal correction minimizes the force to the TMJ and properly aligns its anatomy to absorb this force without breakdown.

An opposite approach from correcting the occlusion at the level of the teeth is to reposition the condyle in the fossa to create radiographic concentric anterior and posterior joint spaces or to protrude the jaw under a displaced disc. This will be discussed with anterior repositioning appliances.

Cognitive awareness is making the patient conscious of oral behavior due to the presence of the OBS, with the goal of reducing muscle activity when teeth contact. A decreased oral volume, altered tongue position, or decreased tactile sensation with the OBS in place may also influence the patient response. Since these nonocclusal factors affect the result of all OBS designs, and this author is unaware of any studies on their specific effects, any comment must await further research.

Placebo effect may also influence OBS therapy when a patient responds positively to a caring and supportive dentist, expects a good result, or is reassured that there is a therapeutic procedure for their problem. Conversely, a bias effect could just as easily be negative for the same reasons: the patient may not like the dentist, may have unrealistic expectations that cannot be met, or may resent the time and cost involved in treatment. Studies have compared nonoccluding with occlusal coverage OBS designs to evaluate the placebo effect.

The superiority of the occluding OBS in reducing signs and symptoms of masticatory muscle problems would show the importance of occlusal control in OBS therapy (Greene and Laskin, 1972; Ekberg, Vallon, and Nilner, 2003; Conti et al., 2006). However, Dao et al. (1994), Cassisi,

McGlynn, and Mahan (1987), and Harada et al. (2006) found equivalent results with the nonoccluding and occluding OBS. Cassisi et al. thought this may be due to altered interocclusal distance by mechanical tongue displacement from the palatal plastic thickness. The placebo effect may influence each patient differently and suggests a benefit of education and emotional support, as an addition to technical excellence.

Disengagement of posterior teeth provides an optimal occlusal scheme that removes force concentration on cuspal interferences during any mandibular movement. Occlusal correction allows TMJ repositioning as the condylar displacement caused by these interferences during mandibular closure is no longer necessary.

The teeth covered by the OBS are protected by the plastic material. The opposing teeth benefit from uniform contact of all teeth on mandibular closure so there is a minimal force on each tooth. The posterior teeth are exposed to only vertical force at closure since they are discluded by the anterior guidance in excursions. It is common to see a decrease in mobility, as well as thermal or pressure sensitivity following OBS insertion.

Occlusal problems occur only when teeth contact and during bruxing and clenching with supranormal forces exceeding mastication, speech, or swallowing. OBS therapy is effective in treating muscle pain by reducing incoordination and hyperactivity associated with protecting teeth from occlusal trauma. Even CR contacts on posterior teeth permit jaw closure without constant compensatory protrusive muscle activity.

Ultra smooth anterior guidance on shallow inclines, separating the posterior teeth, dramatically minimizes the effort that muscles can exert since they have no occlusal interferences to work against. Even with pure clenching, there is equal distribution of force and no need to reposition the jaw to equalize forces on teeth. Dao and Lavigne (1998) questioned whether tooth contacts caused muscle pain since the teeth actually contact for a very limited time of the day. This concern does not address the chronic contraction of the active lateral pterygoid that is programmed to avoid closure on occlusal interferences when it should be inactive during elevator muscle function. Only when the condyles can go to their braced position in CR can this muscle relax during mandibular closure. This critical muscle is deep to the masseter muscle and zygoma and difficult to examine with EMG or ultrasound.

Clinical research and current knowledge of anatomy and biomechanics support the correction of destructive occlusal contacts and their effect on the comfort, function, and integrity of the stomatognathic system. There is no literature describing a benefit to structural breakdown or discomfort from uncontrolled occlusal force. There is no current way to quantify how placebo effect, decreased oral volume, altered tongue space, decreased tactile sensitivity, or passive stretch from the OBS thickness could affect each patient. OBS therapy affects all patients on biomechanical, neurosensory, and emotional levels, combining to form a varied and individual response.

OCCLUSAL BITE SPLINT THERAPY AND SLEEP BRUXISM

Solberg, Clark, and Rugh (1975) found a dramatic reduction of nocturnal masseter muscle EMG activity with maxillary OBS therapy in 8 patients with sleep bruxism (SB). Muscle activity reverted to pretreatment levels after OBS therapy.

Sheikoleslam, Holmgren, and Riise (1986) studied temporal and masseter activity in 31 patients with functional disorders and SB. OBS therapy reduced signs and symptoms of the functional disorders and elevator muscle postural activity. They concluded that OBS therapy is a beneficial symptomatic treatment of the stomatognathic system that facilitates functional analysis and occlusal adjustment.

Hamada et al. (1982) studied 15 bruxists and 20 healthy controls for the effect of OBS therapy on the masseter and temporalis muscles. The steep voltage/tension curves typical of SB became more gentle and similar to healthy subjects after maxillary OBS therapy. This indicated that OBS therapy reduced muscle hyperactivity and restored the resting condition.

Pierce and Gale (1988) studied 100 subjects for the effect of OBS therapy, diurnal and nocturnal biofeedback, and massed negative practice (clenching to the point of discomfort). Compared to controls, the EMG measured frequency and duration of SB decreased only for the nocturnal biofeedback and OBS therapy groups. SB activity returned to baseline levels when treatment was withdrawn.

Clark et al. (1979) measured the masseter activity of 25 patients with myofascial pain dysfunction before, during, and after OBS therapy. Fifty-two percent of patients had decreased nocturnal masseter EMG activity, 24% had no change, and 20% had an increase with treatment. Ninety-two percent returned to pretreatment EMG levels after the removal of the OBS. The majority of patients showed improvement of symptoms even with increased nocturnal EMG levels.

Okkerse et al. (2002) evaluated 21 bruxist patients and 5 controls with an anterior bite plane that did not cover the premolars and molars. They found a significant decrease in nocturnal parafunctional activity of the masseters and anterior temporalis muscles.

Mejias and Mehta (1982) evaluated the effect of either full coverage OBS or an anterior coverage Hawley appliance on SB with a bruxism monitoring device. This was a 0.02-inch colored vacuform plastic appliance that shows wear. Both designs reduced SB significantly and eliminated pain.

Kydd and Daly (1985) evaluated 10 bruxists and 10 controls for the effect of a maxillary OBS. They measured bilateral masseter EMG activity, electrocardiogram (EKG), and body movement. Both bruxists and controls did some nocturnal bruxing. Compared to the above cumulative EMG activity studies, they were able to measure the duration of the SB event. Bruxers clenched for a mean duration of 11.4 minutes and nonbruxers 3.1 minutes. Bruxers had a unilateral and sequential muscle contraction, and clenchers had simultaneous bilateral contractions. OBS therapy did not reduce muscle hyperactivity during SB.

Van der Zaag et al. (2005) used a polysomnographic study (PSG) of twenty-one patients to evaluate the effect of occlusal or palatal coverage OBS designs on SB. They found that neither design affected SB as some patients had increased, decreased, or experienced no change in SB variables. PSG relates SB to sleep, unlike questionnaires, EMG recordings, or evaluation of tooth wear.

Dube, et al. (2004) studied 9 SB patients with PSG for the effect of OBS therapy with occlusal or palatal coverage. Both oral devices showed an equivalent reduction in the number of SB episodes per hour, the number of SB bursts per hour, and the number of episodes with grinding noise.

SB studies with advanced technology continue to yield contradictory results on the effects of OBS therapy. Similar to research on the alteration of occlusion, the dentist should consider these studies with what is known about the effect of forces and the anatomy and pathophysiology of the stomatognathic system. Long-term OBS therapy is accepted to prevent dental attrition. Many but not all studies show additional relief of masticatory muscle hyperactivity and pain. Providing an optimal occlusion is crucial to control muscle forces during mandibular contact and displacement from interfering teeth. This remains true whether SB is due to these contacts or if SB is a central nervous system event creating heavy forces on these teeth.

ANTERIOR REPOSITIONING APPLIANCES

Anterior repositioning appliances (ARA) are directive OBSs, placed on the either the maxillary or mandibular arch that protrude the mandible forward and maintain the condyle in an improved relation with the TMJ disc (figs. 9.24a, 9.24b, and 9.24c). They can be used with patients with displaced discs that reduce (disc realigns with the condyle during protrusion, DDw/R) and don't reduce (disc remains displaced during protrusion, DDw/oR).

Roberts et al. (1986) performed arthrograms on 222 TMJs and found that joint clicking is not necessarily a reducing disc, and the cause and timing of sounds are not clinically diagnostic. There were 13 patients with closing clicks in the nonreducing group. They concluded that in absence of pain and major mechanical dysfunction, clicking alone does not justify treatment. They recommended ARA only after thorough objective evaluation of the type of internal derangement.

Simmons and Gibbs (1995) evaluated 30 patients before and after insertion of a maxillary ARA. MRI showed recapture in 96% of reducing displacements but no recapture in partially or nonreducing joints. All ARAs produced significant pain relief. They stated that MRI is required for patients whose treatment is influenced by disc position; however, MRI studies may differ over time in some patients.

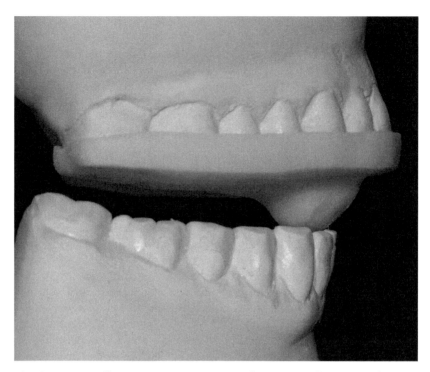

Fig. 9.24a. Maxillary anterior repositioning appliance (ARA) showing initial contact with anterior teeth on closure.

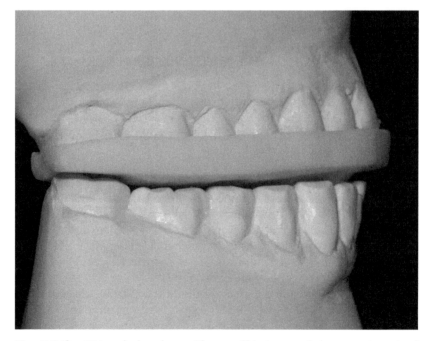

Fig. 9.24b. ARA on further closure (The mandible is protruded to a predetermined condyle/fossa relationship. The acrylic resin ramp guides contact during closure and excursions.).

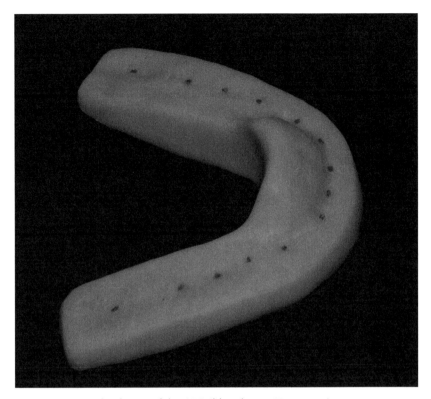

Fig. 9.24c. Occlusal view of the ARA (blue dots = CR contacts).

Kurita et al. (1998) found that 42 of 47 joints that exhibited painful click-ing (DDw/R) were recaptured by the mandibular ARA as shown by MRI. The amount of protrusion of the ARA was determined by clinical resolu-tion of the click.

Lundh et al. (1985) studied 70 patients with pain and dysfunction of the masticatory system and reciprocal clicking. ARA reduced pain during chewing, rest, and protrusion and eliminated reciprocal clicking at six weeks. Clicking returned after the ARA was discontinued. Flat plane occlu-sal splint with group function in lateral excursion decreased joint tender-ness but did not affect clicking or muscle tenderness. The control group showed increased muscle tenderness and the clicking remained.

Chen, Boulton, and Gage (1995) examined 7 patients with MRI after CR OBS therapy. The 3 patients with DDw/R and DDw/oR had improved jaw movement and remission of pain without disc recapture.

Visser, McCarroll, and Naeije (1992) found that an ARA (3 mm pro-truded mandibular position from CR) decreased the activity of the tempo-ralis muscles more than an OBS in CR.

Anderson, Schulte, and Goodkind (1985) compared a CR OBS with canine guidance and a maxillary ARA (in combination with a mandibular segmental appliance) on 20 patients with reciprocal clicking. The repositioning appliances produced significant objective and subjective improvement in the dysfunction of patients with DDw/R, while the CR OBS did not.

Williamson (2005) treated 464 internal derangement patients with a nighttime ARA and a daytime mandibular segmental appliance. After the patient was symptom free, the ARA was reshaped into a CR OBS. After three to five years, 90% of patients reported to be pain free and functionally satisfactory. He recommended use of a CR OBS if there are no signs of disc displacement.

Moloney and Howard (1986) treated 241 patients with disc displacement with an ARA for three to four months and then reshaped it to a CR OBS. After three years, 36% were successfully treated. They noted that if clinical exam shows an anterior displaced disc with late reduction or no reduction, then the chance that the disc is distorted and permanently displaced is high. ARA is contraindicated in these patients and a CR OBS should be used. Patients who had pain on trying to "walk the disc back" to CR require stabilization in the protruded comfortable position by extensive restoration, overlay appliance, orthodontics, or orthognathic surgery.

Okeson (1988) treated 25 patients with disc displacement with eight weeks of continuous ARA use that was then reshaped to a CR OBS. TMJ sounds were relieved one-third of the time with ARA and "step-back" procedures. Pain continued 25% of the time. Eighty percent of patients thought treatment was successful, and 33% sought additional treatment. Okeson concluded that painful joint sounds or progression of joint dysfunction is an indication to treat, and nonpainful unchanging joint sounds do not require treatment. Adaptation of the disc (fibrosis of innervated tissue) is encouraged by the anterior repositioned condyle.

Okeson (1991) stated that during the step-back procedure, when reshaping the ARA to a CR OBS, the disc does not return with the condyle into the fossa. Instead, the condyle returns to the fossa and articulates with retrodiscal tissue. If this tissue has adapted, then loading occurs without pain. He also noted that the majority of patients can be returned to their original occlusal position after ARA, without a permanent posterior open bite. ARA could aggravate DDw/oR by pushing the disc more anteriorly. He recommended ARA use for the short term (four to eight weeks) to avoid pressure from the condyle on traumatized, inflamed retrodiscal tissue. CR OBS therapy after this may be enough for symptomatic relief. The OBS can reduce muscle activity and force to the retrodiscal tissues and should be used instead of ARA if it reduces symptoms.

All ARAs create a posterior open bite due to mandibular protrusion. If that treatment position is chosen, the contacting anterior teeth cannot provide vertical support and stability to the mandible, and force must be redistributed to posterior teeth, requiring dental treatment to establish a posterior occlusion. Even after this is achieved, the lateral pterygoid must remain in a constant contracted state and the condyle contacts the incline of the articular eminence, which is not a stable relationship. If the condyle returns toward the most superior position in the fossa (CR), then the mandible would arc from a more distal axis and occlusal contact would occur on the most posterior tooth. Simmons (personal communication, 2009) stated that pain in the lateral pterygoid from constant contraction is not a clinical problem. The patient is retrained to a new habitual occlusion (established by orthodontics or restoration) with constant use of the ARA at night to maintain the condylar position, without premature contact on the most distal tooth.

ARA therapy has been effective in reducing pain and clicking in DDw/R. It is not a simple therapy, and it is not indicated with DDw/oR. It requires imaging to initially position the condyle and creates a posterior open bite that must be treated with comprehensive dentistry. Reshaping the ARA into a CR OBS has not been predictable. An OBS that allows the condyle to go to CR and provides an optimal occlusion should be used if it reduces symptoms.

CONCLUSION

The stomatognathic system is composed of strong, resilient, and durable structures. For this system to last a lifetime, all of its components must function harmoniously. Coordinated muscle activity and a proper occlusion are required to preserve teeth during function. Force levels of mastication or oral habits must remain within physiologic limits for muscles and TMJs to repair themselves and preserve the integrity of the system. The dentist is the only professional who is trained to diagnose and treat problems from destructive forces exceeding the system's ability to maintain itself. Mastering OBS therapy is a fundamental step in building a practice that can provide optimal occlusion for predictable equilibration and restorative dentistry.

REFERENCES

Academy of Prosthodontics. (2005). The glossary of prosthodontic terms. *Journal of Prosthetic Dentistry*, Vol. 94, pp. 1–92.

Al Quran, F.A.M., and Lyons, M.F. (1999). The immediate effect of hard and soft splints on the EMG activity of the masseter and temporalis muscles. *Journal of Oral Rehabilitation*, Vol. 26, pp. 559–563.

Anderson, G.C., Schulte, J.K., Goodkind, R.J. (1985). Comparative study of two treatment methods for internal derangement of the temporomandibular joint. *Journal of Prosthetic Dentistry*, Vol. 53, pp. 392–397.

Barker, D.K. (2004). Occlusal interferences and temporomandibular dysfunction. *General Dentistry*, Vol. 52, pp. 56–61.

Beard, C.C., and Clayton, J.A. (1980). Effects of occlusal splint therapy on TMJ dysfunction. *Journal of Prosthetic Dentistry*, Vol. 44, pp. 324–335.

Becker, I., Tarantola, G., Zambrano, J., et al. (1999). Effect of a prefabricated anterior bite stop on electromyographic activity of masticatory muscles. *Journal of Prosthetic Dentistry*, Vol. 82, pp. 22–26.

Bonfante, G., Ramos, L., and Bonfante, E.A. (2003). Restoration of canine guidance on an occlusal splint using amalgam: A clinical report. *Journal of Prosthetic Dentistry*, Vol. 90, pp. 420–423.

Braem, M., Lambrechts, P., and Vanherle, G. (1982). Stress-induced cervical lesions. *Journal of Prosthetic Dentistry*, Vol. 67, pp. 718–722.

Carlsson, G.E., Ingervall, B., and Kocak, G. (1979). Effect of increasing vertical dimension on the masticatory system in subjects with natural teeth. *Journal of Prosthetic Dentistry*, Vol. 41, pp. 284–289.

Carraro, J.J., and Caffesse, R.G. (1978). Effect of occlusal splints on TMJ symptomatology. *Journal of Prosthetic Dentistry*, Vol. 40, pp. 563–566.

Cassisi, J.E., McGlynn, F.D., and Mahan, P.E. (1987). Occlusal splint effects on nocturnal bruxing: An emerging paradigm and some early results. *Journal of Craniomandibular Practice*, Vol. 5, pp. 65–68.

Chen, C.W., Boulton, J.L., and Gage, J.P. (1995). Effect of splint therapy in TMJ dysfunction: A study using magnetic resonance imaging. *Australian Dental Journal*, Vol. 40, pp. 71–78.

Clark, G.T. (1984a). A critical evaluation of orthopedic interocclusal appliance therapy: Design, theory, and overall effectiveness. *Journal of the American Dental Association*, Vol. 108, pp. 359–364.

Clark, G.T. (1984b). A critical evaluation of orthopedic interocclusal appliance therapy: Effectiveness for specific symptoms. *Journal of the American Dental Association*, Vol. 108, pp. 364–368.

Clark, G.T., Beemsterboer, P.L., Solberg W.K., et al. (1979). Nocturnal electromyographic Evaluation of myofascial pain dysfunction in patients undergoing splint therapy. *Journal of the American Dental Association*, Vol. 99, pp. 607–611.

Conti, P.C.R., Santos, C.N., Kogawa, E.M., et al. (2006). The treatment of painful temporomandibular joint clicking with oral splints. *Journal of the American Dental Association*, Vol. 137, pp. 1008–1014.

Dao, T.T., and Lavigne, G.J. (1998). Oral splints: The crutches for temporomandibular disorders and bruxism? *Critical Reviews in Oral Biology and Medicine*, Vol. 9, pp. 345–361.

Dao, T.T., Lavigne, G.C., Charbonneau, A., et al. (1994). The efficacy of oral splints in the treatment of myofascial pain of the jaw muscles: A controlled clinical trial. *Pain*, Vol. 56, pp. 85–94.

Dawson, P.E. (1973). Temporomandibular joint pain-dysfunction problems can be solved. *Journal of Prosthetic Dentistry*, Vol. 29, pp. 100–112.

Dawson, P.E. (1985). Optimum TMJ condyle position in clinical practice. *International Journal of Periodontics and Restorative Dentistry*, Vol. 5, pp. 10–31.

Dawson, P.E. (1989). *Evaluation, Diagnosis, and Treatment of Occlusal Problems*. 2nd Edition. St. Louis: Mosby.

Dube, C., Rompre, P.H., Manzini, C., et al. (2004). Quantitative polygraphic controlled study on efficacy and safety of oral splint devices in tooth-grinding subjects. *Journal of Dental Research*, Vol. 83, pp. 398–403.

Dyer, E.H. (1973). Importance of a stable maxillomandibular relation. *Journal of Prosthetic Dentistry*, Vol. 30, pp. 241–251.

Ekberg, E.C., Vallon, D., and Nilner, M. (2003). The efficacy of appliance therapy in patients with temporomandibular disorders mainly of myogenous origin. A randomized, controlled, short-term trial. *Journal of Orofacial Pain*, Vol. 17, pp. 133–139.

Emshoff, R., and Bertram, S. (1998). The short-term effect of stabilization-type splints on local cross-sectional dimensions of muscles of the head and neck. *Journal of Prosthetic Dentistry*, Vol. 80, pp. 457–461.

Fitins, D., and Sheikholeslam, A. (1993). Effect of canine guidance of maxillary occlusal splint on level of activation of masticatory muscles. *Swedish Dental Journal*, Vol. 17, pp. 235–241.

Fu, A.S., Mehta, N.R., Forgione, A.G., et al. (2003). Maxillomandibular relationship in TMD patients before and after short-term flat plane bite plate therapy. *Journal of Craniomandibular Practice*, Vol. 21, pp. 172–178.

Gibbs, C.H., Mahan, P.E., Wilkinson, T.M., et al. (1984). EMG activity of the superior belly of the lateral pterygoid muscle in relation to other jaw muscles. *Journal of Prosthetic Dentistry*, Vol. 51, pp. 691–702.

Graham, G.S., and Rugh, J.D. (1988). Maxillary splint occlusal guidance patterns and electromyographic activity of the jaw-closing muscles. *Journal of Prosthetic Dentistry*, Vol. 59, pp. 73–77.

Grant, D.A., Stern, I.B., Everett, F.G. (1972). *Orban's Periodontics*, 4th ed. St. Louis: Mosby.

Greene, C.S., and Laskin, D.M. (1972). Splint therapy for the myofascial pain-dysfunction (MPD). syndrome: A comparative study. *Journal of the American Dental Association*, Vol. 84, pp. 624–628.

Grippo, J.O. (1991). Abfractions: A new classification of hard tissue lesions of teeth. *Journal of Esthetic Dentistry*, Vol. 3, pp. 14–18.

Hamada, T., Kotani, H., Kawazoe, Y., et al. (1982). Effect of occlusal splints on the EMG activity of masseter and temporalis muscles in bruxism with clinical symptoms. *Journal of Oral Rehabilitation*, Vol. 9, pp. 119–123.

Harada, T., Ichiki, R., Tsukiyama, Y., et al. (2006). The effect of oral splint devices on sleep bruxism: A 6-week observation with an ambulatory electromyographic recording device. *Journal of Oral Rehabilitation*, Vol. 33, pp. 482–488.

Harrel, S.K. (2006). Is there an association between occlusion and periodontal destruction? *Journal of the American Dental Association*, Vol. 137, pp. 1380–1392.

Haywood, V.B., and Powe, A. (1998). Using double-poured alginate impressions to fabricate bleaching trays. *Operative Dentistry*, Vol. 23, pp. 128–131.

Hellsing, G. (1984). Functional adaptation to changes in vertical dimension. *Journal of Prosthetic Dentistry*, Vol. 52, pp. 867–870.

Humsi, A.N.K., Naeije, M., Hippe, J A , et al. (1989). The immediate effect of a stabilization splint on the muscular symmetry in the masseter and anterior temporal muscles of patients with a craniomandibular disorder. *Journal of Prosthetic Dentistry*, Vol. 62, pp. 339–343.

Israel, H.A., Diamond, B., Saed-Nejad, F., et al. (1999). The relationship between parafunctional masticatory activity and arthroscopically diagnosed temporomandibular joint pathology. *Journal of Oral and Maxillofacial Surgery*, Vol. 57, pp. 1034–1039.

Ito, T., Gibbs, C.H., Marguelles-Bonnet, R., et al. (1986). Loading on the temporomandibular joints with five occlusal conditions. *Journal of Prosthetic Dentistry*, Vol. 56, pp. 478–484.

Jimenez, I. (1987). Dental stability and maximal masticatory muscle activity. *Journal of Oral Rehabilitation*, Vol. 14, pp. 591–598.

Johnston, L.E., and EICO Orthodontic Study Group of Ohio. (1988). Gnathologic assessment of centric slides in post-retention orthodontic patients. *Journal of Prosthetic Dentistry*, Vol. 60, pp. 712–715.

Juniper, R.P. (1984). Temporomandibular joint dysfunction: A theory based upon electromyographic studies of the lateral pterygoid muscle. *British Journal of Oral and Maxillofacial Surgery*, Vol. 22, pp. 1–8.

Kerstein, R.B., and Farrell, S. (1990). Treatment of myofascial pain dysfunction syndrome with occlusal equilibration. *Journal of Prosthetic Dentistry*, Vol. 63, pp. 695–700.

Kerstein, R.B., and Wright, N.R. (1991). Electromyographic and computer analyses of patients suffering from chronic myofascial pain-dysfunction syndrome: Before and after treatment with immediate complete anterior guidance development. *Journal of Prosthetic Dentistry*, Vol. 66, pp. 677–686.

Kurita, H., Ikeda, K., and Kurashina, K. (2000). Evaluation of a stabilization splint on occlusal force in patients with masticatory muscle disorders. *Journal of Oral Rehabilitation*, Vol. 27, pp. 79–82.

Kurita, H., Kurashina, K., Baba, H., et al. (1998). Evaluation of disk capture with a splint repositioning appliance: Clinical and critical assessment with MR imaging. *Oral Surgery, Oral Medicine, Oral Pathology, Oral Radiology and Endodontics*, Vol. 85, pp. 377–380.

Kydd, W.L., and Daly, C. (1985). *Duration of* nocturnal tooth contacts during bruxing. *Journal of Prosthetic Dentistry*, Vol. 53, pp. 717–721.

Lee, W.C., and Eakle, W.S. (1984). Possible role of tensile stress in the etiology of cervical erosive lesions of teeth. *Journal of Prosthetic Dentistry*, Vol. 52, pp. 374–380.

Lee, W.C., and Eakle, W.S. (1996). Stress-induced cervical lesions: Review of advances in the past 10 years. *Journal of Prosthetic Dentistry*, Vol. 75, pp. 487–494.

Lous, I. (1978). Treatment of TMJ syndrome by pivots. *Journal of Prosthetic Dentistry*, Vol. 40, pp. 179–182.

Lundeen HC. (1974). Centric relation records: The effect of muscle action. *Journal of Prosthetic Dentistry*, 31, 244–251.

Lundh, H., Westesson, P.L., Kopp, S., et al. (1985). Anterior repositioning splint in the treatment of temporomandibular joints reciprocal clicking: Comparison with a flat occlusal splint and an untreated control group. *Oral Surgery, Oral Medicine, Oral Pathology, Oral Radiology, and Endodontics*, Vol. 60, pp. 131–136.

Lytle, J.D. (2001). Occlusal disease revisited: Part II. *International Journal of Periodontics and Restorative Dentistry*, Vol. 21, pp. 273–279.

Mahan, P.E., Wilkinson, T.M., Gibbs, C.H., et al. (1983). Superior and inferior bellies of the lateral pterygoid muscle: EMG activity at basic jaw positions. *Journal of Prosthetic Dentistry*, Vol. 50, pp. 710–718.

Manns, A., Chan, C., and Miralles, R. (1987). Influence of group function and canine guidance on electromyographic activity of elevator muscles. *Journal of Prosthetic Dentistry*, Vol. 57, pp. 494–501.

Manns, A., Miralles, R., Santander, H., et al. (1983). Influence of the vertical dimension in the treatment of myofascial pain-dysfunction syndrome. *Journal of Prosthetic Dentistry*, Vol. 59, pp. 700–709.

McGuire, M.K., and Nunn, M.E. (1996). Prognosis versus actual outcome: III. The effectiveness of clinical parameters in accurately predicting tooth survival. *Journal of Periodontology*, Vol. 67, pp. 666–674.

McKee, J.R. (1997). Comparing condylar position repeatability for standardized versus nonstandardized methods of achieving centric relation. *Journal of Prosthetic Dentistry*, Vol. 77, pp. 280–284.

McKee, J.R. (2005). Comparing condylar positions achieved through bimanual manipulation to condylar positions achieved through masticatory muscle contraction against an anterior deprogrammer: A pilot study. *Journal of Prosthetic Dentistry*, Vol. 94, pp. 389–393.

McNeill, C. (1985). The optimum temporomandibular joint condyle position in clinical practice. *International Journal of Periodontics and Restorative Dentistry*, Vol. 5, pp. 53–77.

Mejias, J.E., and Mehta, N.R. (1982). Subjective and objective evaluation of bruxing patients undergoing short-term splint therapy. *Journal of Oral Rehabilitation*, Vol. 9, pp. 279–289.

Moloney, F., and Howard, J.A. (1986). Internal derangements of the temporomandibular joint: III. Anterior repositioning splint therapy. *Australian Dental Journal*, Vol. 31, pp. 30–39.

Mongini, F. (1972). Remodeling of the mandibular condyle in the adult and its relationship to the condition of the dental arches. *Acta Anatomica*, Vol. 82, pp. 437–453.

Mongini, F. (1980). Condylar remodeling after occlusal therapy. *Journal of Prosthetic Dentistry*, Vol. 43, pp. 568–577.

Nitzan, D.W. (1994). Intra-articular pressure in the functioning human temporomandibular joint and its alteration by uniform elevation of the occlusal plane. *Journal of Oral and Maxillofacial Surgery*, Vol. 52, pp. 671–679.

Nitzan, D.W. (2001). The process of lubrication impairment and its involvement in temporomandibular joint disc displacement: A theoretical concept. *Journal Oral Maxillofacial Surgery*, Vol. 59, pp. 36–45.

Nitzan, D.W., and Marmary, Y. (1997). The "anchored disc phenomenon": A proposed etiology for sudden-onset, severe and persistent closed lock of the temporomandibular joint. *Journal Oral Maxillofacial Surgery*, Vol. 55, pp. 797–802.

Noble, W.H. (1975). Anteroposterior position of "Myo-Monitor centric." *Journal of Prosthetic Dentistry*, Vol. 33, pp. 398–402.

Nunn, M.E., and Harrel, S.K. (2001a). The effect of occlusal discrepancies on periodontitis: 1. Relationship of initial occlusal discrepancies to initial clinical parameters. *Journal of Periodontology*, Vol. 72, pp. 485–494.

Nunn, M.E., and Harrel, S.K. (2001b). The effect of occlusal discrepancies on periodontitis: 2. Relationship of occlusal treatment to progession of periodontal disease. *Journal of Periodontology*, Vol. 72, pp. 495–505.

Oh, T.J., et al. (2002). The causes of early implant bone loss: Myth or science. *Journal of Periodontology*, Vol. 73, pp. 322–333.

Okeson, J.P. (1987). The effects of hard and soft occlusal splints on nocturnal bruxism. *Journal of the American Dental Association*, Vol. 114, pp. 788–791.

Okeson, J.P. (1988). Long-term treatment of disk-interference disorders of the temporomandibular joint with anterior repositioning occlusal splints. *Journal of Prosthetic Dentistry*, Vol. 60, pp. 611–616.

Okeson, J.P. (1991). Nonsurgical management of disc-interference disorders. *Dental Clinic of North America*, Vol. 35, pp. 29–51.

Okeson, J.P., Dickson, J.L., Kemper, J.T. (1982). The influence of assisted mandibular movement on the incidence of nonworking contact. *Journal of Prosthetic Dentistry*, Vol. 4, pp. 174–177.

Okeson, J.P., Kemper, J.T., Moody, P.M. (1982). A study of the use of occlusion splints in the treatment of acute and chronic patients with craniomandibular disorders. *Journal of Prosthetic Dentistry*, Vol. 48, pp. 708–712.

Okkerse, W., Brebels, A., De Deyn, P.P., et al. (2002). Influence of a bite-plane according to Jeanmonod, on bruxism activity during sleep. *Journal of Oral Rehabilitation*, Vol. 29, pp. 980–985.

Pierce, C.J., and Gale, E.N. (1988). A comparison of different treatments for nocturnal bruxism. *Journal of Dental Research*, Vol. 67, pp. 597–601.

Radu, J., Marandici, M., and Hottel, T.L. (2004). The effect of clenching on condylar position: A vector analysis model. *Journal of Prosthetic Dentistry*, Vol. 91, pp. 171–179.

Ramfjord, S.P., and Ash, M.M. (1994). Reflections on the Michigan occlusal splint. *Journal of Oral Rehabilitation*, Vol. 21, pp. 491–500.

Rehany, A., and Stern, N. (1981). The modified Hawley occlusal splint. *Journal of Prosthetic Dentistry*, Vol. 45, pp. 536–541.

Remien, J.C., and Ash, M.M. (1974). "Myo-Monitor centric": An evaluation. *Journal of Prosthetic Dentistry*, Vol. 31, pp. 137–145.

Roberts, C.A., Tallents, R.H., Katzberg, R.W., et al. (1986). Clinical and arthrographic evaluation of temporomandibular joint sounds. *Oral Surgery, Oral Medicine, Oral Pathology, Oral Radiology, and Endodontics*, Vol. 62, pp. 373–376.

Roth, R.H. (1973). Temporomandibular pain-dysfunction and occlusal relationships. *Angle Orthodontist*, Vol. 43, pp. 136–153.

Rugh, J.D., and Drago, C.J. (1981). Vertical dimension: A study of clinical rest position and jaw muscle activity. *Journal of Prosthetic Dentistry*, Vol. 45, pp. 670–675.

Rugh, J.D., Graham, G.S., Smith, J.C., et al. (1989). Effects of canine versus molar occlusal splint guidance on nocturnal bruxism and craniomandibular symptomatology. *Journal of Crandiomandibular Disorders: Facial and Oral Pain*, Vol. 3, pp. 203–210.

Schwartz, R., Kudyba, P., and Martine, J.O. (1986). Use criteria for occlusal equilibration and splint therapy: II. Maxillary and mandibular midlines as points of reference. *Clinical Preventive Dentistry*, Vol. 8, pp. 24–29.

Scopel, V., Costa, G.S.A., and Urias, D. (2005). An electromyographic study of masseter and anterior temporalis muscles in extra-articular myogenous TMJ pain patients compared to an asymptomatic normal population. *Journal of Craniomandibular Practice*, Vol. 23, pp. 194–203.

Sears, V.H. (1956). Occlusal pivots. *Journal of Prosthetic Dentistry*, Vol. 6, pp. 332–338.

Sheikoleslam, A., Holmgren, K., and Riise, C. (1986). A clinical and electromyographic study of the long-term effects of an occlusal splint on the temporal and masseter muscles in patients with functional disorders and nocturnal bruxism. *Journal of Oral Rehabilitation*, Vol. 13, pp. 137–145.

Shupe, R.J., Mohamed, S.E., Christensen, L.V., et al. (1984). Effects of occlusal guidance on jaw muscle activity. *Journal of Prosthetic Dentistry*, Vol. 51, pp. 811–818.

Simmons, H.C., and Gibbs, S.J. (1995). Recapture of temporomandibular joint disks using anterior repositioning appliances: An MRI study. *Journal of Craniomandibular Practice*, Vol. 13, pp. 227–237.

Solberg, W.K., Clark, J.T., and Rugh, J.D. (1975). Nocturnal electromyographic evaluation of bruxism patients undergoing short-term splint therapy. *Journal of Oral Rehabilitation*, Vol. 2, pp. 215–223.

Solow, R.A. (1999). The anterior acrylic resin platform and centric relation verification: A clinical report. *Journal of Prosthetic Dentistry*, Vol. 81, pp. 255–257.

Solow, R.A. (2005). Equilibration of a progressive anterior open occlusal relationship: A clinical report. *Journal of Craniomandibular Practice*, Vol. 23, pp. 229–238.

Stegenga, B. (2000). Osteoarthritis of the temporomandibular joint organ and its relationship to disc displacement. *Journal of Orofacial Pain*, Vol. 15, pp. 193–205.

Steigenga, J., Al-Shammari, K., Misch, C., et al. (2004). Effects of implant thread geometry on percentage of osseointegration and resistance to reverse torque in the tibia of rabbits. *Journal of Periodontology*, Vol. 75, pp. 133–141.

Strohaver, R.A. (1972). A comparison of articulator mountings made with centric relation and myocentric position records. *Journal of Prosthetic Dentistry*, Vol. 28, pp. 379–390.

Tarantola, G.J., Becker, I.M., Gremillion, H. (1997). The reproducibility of centric relation: A clinical approach. *Journal of the American Dental Association*, Vol. 128, pp. 1245–1251.

Tarantola, G.J., Becker, I.M., Gremillion, H., et al. (1998) The effectiveness of equilibration in the improvement of signs and symptoms in the stomato-gnathic system. *International Journal of Periodontics and Restorative Dentistry*, Vol. 18, pp. 595–603.

Tsuga, K., Akagawa, Y., Sakaguchi, R., et al. (1989). A short-term evaluation of the effectiveness of stabilization-type occlusal splint therapy for specific symptoms of temporomandibular joint dysfunction syndrome. *Journal of Prosthetic Dentistry*, Vol. 61, pp. 610–613.

Van der Zaag, J., Lobbezoo, F., Wicks, D.J., et al. (2005). Controlled assessment of the efficacy of occlusal stabilization splints on sleep bruxism. *Journal of Orofacial Pain*, Vol. 19, pp. 151–158.

Visser, A., McCarroll, R.S., and Naeije, M. (1992). Masticatory muscle activity in different jaw relations during submaximal clenching efforts. *Journal of Dental Research*, Vol. 71, pp. 372–378.

Wang, M.Q., He, J.J., Li, G., et al. (2008). The effect of physiological nonbalanced occlusion on the thickness of the temporomandibular joint disc: A pilot autopsy study. *The Journal of Prosthetic Dentistry*, Vol. 98, pp. 148–152.

Wessberg, G.A., Epker, B.N., Elliott, A.C. (1983). Comparison of mandibular rest positions induced by phonetic, transcutaneous electrical stimulation, and masticatory electromyography. *Journal of Prosthetic Dentistry*, Vol. 49, pp. 100–105.

Widmer, C.G., Lund, J.P., Feine, J.S. (1990). Evaluation of diagnostic tests for TMD. *Journal of the California Dental Association*, Vol. 18, pp. 53–60.

Wilkerson, D.C. (2009). A clinician's guide to occlusal splint therapy. *Vistas*, Vol. 2, pp. 8–20.

Williamson, E.H. (2005). Temporomandibular dysfunction and repositioning splint therapy. *Progress in Orthodontics*, Vol. 2, pp. 206–213.

Williamson, E.H., Evans, D.L., Barton, W.A., et al. (1977). The effect of bite plane use on terminal hinge axis location. *Angle Orthodontist*, Vol. 47, pp. 25–33.

Williamson, E.H., and Lundquist, D.O. (1983). Anterior guidance: Its effect on electromyographic activity of the temporal and masseter muscles. *Journal of Prosthetic Dentistry*, Vol. 49, pp. 816–823.

Yamada, K., Hanada, K., Fukui, T., et al. (2001). Condylar bony change and self-reported parafunctional habits in prospective orthognathic surgery patients with temporomandibular disorders. *Oral Surgery, Oral Pathology, Oral Medicine, Oral Radiology, and Endodontics*, Vol. 92, pp. 265–271.

Occlusal Equilibration and the Diagnostic Workup

Irwin M. Becker, DDS

To reorganize a patient's occlusion, it is imperative that the clinician first perform a comprehensive evaluation including articulated casts, mounted with a reasonable facebow and a verified centric relation (CR) record. The verification includes matching first point of contact on the casts with intra-oral markings, as well as matching excursive disclusive patterns by appropriately dialing in articulator condylar settings. These verifications usually follow occlusal bite splint therapy.

One should also know what relationships exist among any signs, symptoms, and subclinical responses that present themselves with the patient in question. If none exist, changing the occlusion might be contra-indicated. In general, the clinician should only equilibrate if there are signs of occlusal instability, but there is one possible exception—the clinician may change the occlusion to make the planned restorative dentistry more predictable.

Once teeth are prepared with occlusal reductions of perhaps 2 mm, one can rationalize that the equilibration has actually begun as the precious, acquired occlusal inclines are wiped away. It has never been shown that these incline contacts can be predictably put back. Thus, the bite has been changed, and this author believes that once the occlusal contacts in an acquired bite are changed, the only contacts available for completing adjustment are the CR arc of closure occlusal contacts.

Prior to beginning any sort of occlusal reorganization, one should recognize the complexity of the specific tasks involved. Occlusal equilibration, while quite reasonable and understandable as a comprehensive thought process, is perhaps the most technically challenging process in its demand

Comprehensive Occlusal Concepts in Clinical Practice, by Irwin M. Becker
© 2011 Blackwell Publishing Ltd.

of hand-eye coordination. Because it is completely irreversible, careful preparation must be made to avoid error.

It would take a complex computer program to make each cut on stone precisely duplicate each cut on tooth structure, both subtractive and additive. As such a program is not currently available, the best preparation is completely visualizing the starting point, finishing point, and entire equilibration process on articulated casts.

The clinician typically needs to return to the original vertical dimension at the time equilibration is finished unless he or she is attempting to increase vertical dimension of occlusion or attempting to close the bite. Grinding can be done on a patient's bite only because, in the new CR arc of closure, there is an open or increased vertical dimension of occlusion (see fig. 10.1.) Otherwise, equilibration techniques would close down the bite, which is not desired in most cases.

Typically, when a patient is hinged in the new CR arc of closure, the first point of contact is open compared with the maximum intercuspal position. In fact, a clinical observation is that the greater the vertical opening is in CR, the easier the subsequent equilibration will be because there is more room to jockey around the cusp-fossa inclinations before closing vertically. Likewise, the most difficult equilibrations tend to be when there is no vertical change between maximum intercuspal position and first point of contact. Often this latter situation requires orthodontics or restorative intervention.

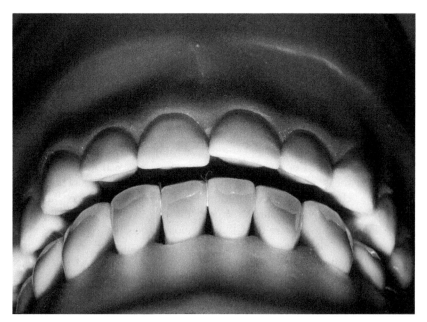

Fig. 10.1. Open or increased vertical dimension of occlusion in centric relation arc of closure.

The clinician needs to recognize exactly when equilibration alone is appropriate and when additional treatment modalities will be required. Understanding of the equilibration process leads to more reasonable decisions about when equilibration alone can be predictably performed.

The other big question that routinely presents itself is whether a reasonable anterior guidance can be obtained through equilibration alone, or whether orthodontics and/or restorative treatment be required. It is precisely this question that has prompted this author to think of all esthetic considerations as a subset of anterior guidance. The thinking being that any time the clinician is asked to improve or change a patient's esthetics, treatment could include comprehensive reorganization of the occlusion to improve not only the smile and appearance but also improve function and diminish any effects of parafunctional activities.

Many detailed decisions during the act of equilibration will be based on esthetic considerations. It is best not to tell the patient about a planned treatment prior to the trial equilibration. Otherwise, the patient might expect a simple equilibration only to find out later that orthodontics will be actually required. This presents a problem for both the patient and dentist.

Going back to the earlier statement that the thought process of equilibration is reasonable and straightforward, it is actually similar to the adjustment of an occlusal bite splint. The objective is to obtain a maximum number of centric stops along the long axis of each occluding tooth during CR arc of closure. Furthermore, the clinician seeks to provide an anterior guidance that is appropriate for the patient in question to solve the puzzle of smile design and to provide immediate posterior disclusion that is characterized by smooth crossover with the least incline that still discludes the rest of the posterior teeth, has no inappropriate distalizing inclines, allows crisp and comfortable phonetics, and is stable and comfortable.

Today we look at the equilibration process as both subtractive and additive. The trial equilibration is thought of as a diagnostic workup in which sometimes stone is removed and sometimes wax is added. The determination of the appropriate sequence involves evaluating the case for what is the biggest part of the problem. If the primary objective is to obtain centric stops and correct the slide from first point of contact, start with CR adjustments. If the greatest need is anterior guidance, then start there. If the biggest concern is esthetics, also start with the guidance. Even if the plan is to start with centric adjustments, take care of the anterior edges early on.

Lower incisal plane irregularities should be addressed early on. Even though esthetic considerations generally force the clinician to evaluate the maxillary anterior set of teeth during the clinical chairside examination, when working up the case on the lab bench with articulated casts, setting up the lower anterior incisal plane takes priority as the first step. This is because the mandible is the moving unit and its incisal edge passes along on the static lingual contours of the maxillary lingual contour. Also, this is because so many factors are actually determined from the character and position of the anterior lower edges. Some of the factors are vertical dimension, quality of edge-to-edge position, and crossover smoothness.

Even before contemplating the steps of actual equilibration, the reader should review the following set of time-proven recommendations:

- Do not equilibrate unless there are signs of occlusal instability.
- Do not equilibrate unless you have verified the diagnosis and verified it is related to occlusal instability.
- Know exactly what CR arc of closure implies and understand the timing to the eventual seating of the condyle.
- Do not equilibrate until you have honed your skills of splint therapy and trial equilibration, and can guide the patient into CR arc of closure or some reasonable treatment position. The literature is replete with studies that indicate the reproducibility of CR arc of closure, as well as the effective use of the anterior deprogrammer. Lucia, 1964; Tarantola, Becker, and Gremillion, 1997; Becker et al., 1999; Karl and Foley, 1999; McKee, 1977, 2005; Solow, 1999; and Williamson et al., 1980, are but a few of the time-tested references.

THE FALLACY OF INSTANT ORTHODONTIC THERAPY

This author would like to take the opportunity to comment on the current trend in avoiding orthodontics when dealing with crooked and malaligned anterior teeth. It is in vogue today to simply put veneer-type restorations on anterior teeth that actually need to be aligned. Veneer systems leave the teeth without proper vertical axial loading capacity, and the interproximal embrasures with a pathologic relationship that leads to difficult flossing. The poor alignment also leads to interproximal papillae that have an improper contour and difficult-to-maintain biologic width in the most susceptible area. Poorly aligned teeth force the restorative dentist to create an artificial labial and interproximal contour. These contours are often severely overcontoured, leading to possible negative effects on the gingival tissues. Furthermore, overcontouring can decrease the longevity of these esthetic restorations and can lead to future unnecessary dentistry.

To skip over orthodontic therapy and suggest inappropriate veneering is actually an affront to our professional integrity. The patient ultimately will make a personal decision, but it is critical that the dentist explain the options fully and discuss the shortcomings of the quick fix in this situation.

RATIONALE OF THE TRIAL EQUILIBRATION

It is important to review at this time why it is essential to perform a trial equilibration (figs. 10.2 and 10.3) prior to doing the actual irreversible

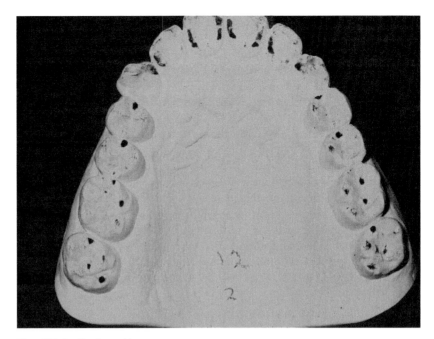

Fig. 10.2. Trial equilibration.

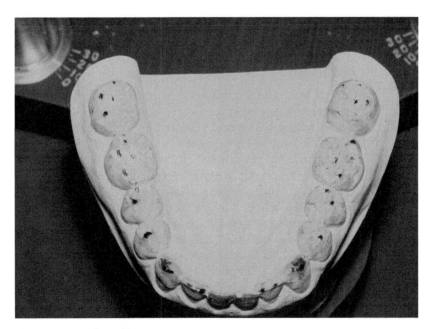

Fig. 10.3. Trial equilibration.

procedure. The clinician needs to know exactly where the end point will be. If the end point is not clearly visualized, the possibility increases of going way too far in reduction. Dentists have been sued because of this error.

On articulated casts, the vertical pin indicates when the original vertical dimension of occlusion is restored. By recording the anterior-most tooth contact that touches in the acquired bite, the clinician will know to return to this contact at the conclusion of the occlusal reorganization. Alternatively, the clinician can return to a reasonable anterior guidance. The clinician needs to ask whether equilibration alone will bring the case down to acceptable anterior guidance or whether additional treatment modalities will be needed. Remember that almost every equilibration starts at an open vertical dimension and must return to original vertical, a predetermined vertical, or at least an acceptable anterior guidance.

THE TEN STEPS OF THE TRIAL EQUILIBRATION

The term *trial equilibration* can be often interchanged with *diagnostic workup* or even *reorganizing the occlusion*. More and more today, the trial equilibration is not simply a take-away procedure. Often, additive wax on the casts or composite restorative material is bonded intraorally.

Step 1: Evaluate Anterior Guidance in Habitual Occlusion

Beware that once the mandible is hinged in the centric relation arc of closure, it becomes quite questionable whether equilibration can return the patient to original vertical or even an acceptable anterior guidance.

The clinician has the opportunity to notice and mark the anterior-most contact in acquired centric. This allows an intraoral reference when it comes to vertical dimension. Generally, the recommended finishing point is when the mouth is returned to this anterior-most tooth contact. Therefore, if the central incisors were touching in maximum intercuspation, they may need to touch again after the equilibration process is finished.

The reason for this is multifold. First, it brings the patient back to approximately the same original vertical dimension of occlusion. This leads to better, more predictable comfort—and stops the muscles from closing down the vertical. If equilibration were to increase the space between the upper and lower anterior teeth, a phonetic problem could result, as well as a discernable difference in proprioception. Also, the intra-arch relationship might be altered sufficiently to cause the patient to notice some unexplainable bad feeling. So, taking phonetics, comfort, and muscle tension into consideration, it is wise and prudent to have in mind this easy-to-recognize finishing point—the anterior-most contact in acquired centric.

An exception to this is when the case has an anterior open bite to begin with. Then, the cuspids or bicuspids will be the reference point instead of the incisors. In this case, the clinician needs to determine if the open bite can be closed sufficiently to bring more anterior teeth into contact, allowing incisal coupling. The clinician needs to evaluate what action will be most appropriate: closing vertical by removing tooth structure, orthodontics, or restorative techniques, or leaving the patient with an open bite. Leaving the patient with an anterior open bite means there will be a compromised guidance that starts with bicuspids and transitions to the cuspids if possible.

On the articulated casts, the clinician sets the vertical pin based on maximum intercuspation and thus is able to evaluate the most appropriate action quite precisely. Unfortunately, there is no intraoral pin.

Step 2A: Evaluate the Amount of Vertical Opening at the First Point of Contact

Contrary to popular opinion, the more open the relationship is at the first point of contact, the easier the equilibration will be to accomplish. This is simply because there will be more room to jockey cusp-fossa shapes and inclines to reach the end point, prior to closing vertical. In fact, the most difficult case to equilibrate is one that does not open at first point of contact. These cases may have a significant slide from the first point to maximum intercuspal position, but because of the lack of well-defined anatomy there is very little vertical separation. Thus, as soon as one starts to grind inclines away, vertical begins to close. Be very careful. These are the occlusal cases that are better corrected with restorative measures to create a more normal anatomy. By taking note of the amount of separation in the beginning, the clinician can avoid a major surprise at the end of the trial equilibration. This author's experience supports the necessity of doing a trial equilibration in cases that do not open at first point of contact.

It should be also noted that not all cases are returned to the original vertical. Some that will be undergoing restorative measures may be purposely increased in vertical dimension because of prosthetic needs. Sometimes there is not enough room for restorative material, or esthetic objectives indicate increasing vertical. In a case that has lost vertical, the diagnostic workup may indicate the need to purposely restore lost vertical. The clinician must always be sure in that case that the vertical has been actually been lost. Attrition, even severe wear, generally does not indicate a loss in vertical dimension. Studies clearly indicate that there almost always is compensatory eruption and alveolar growth. Studies over 20 years indicate that even when the teeth have been worn down to the gingival unit, the measured vertical dimension of occlusion has stayed the same (Begg, 1954; Berry and Poole, 1976; Crothers, 1992; Crothers and Sandham, 1993; Kaifu et al., 2008; Murphy, 1959; Sicher, 1953; Whittaker et al., 1985).

The true lost vertical case is almost always a neglected, untreated patient with either no posterior teeth or posterior teeth that have collapsed forward due to periodontal disease. This loss has occurred more quickly than the attempted physiologic compensation can maintain. Also, this true-loss case has splayed maxillary anteriors, indicating a lack of any reasonable vertical stops.

An important point to remember is that whenever vertical opening is planned, the clinician should never open past the patient's acquired free-way space. Where the violation of free-way space has been observed, the speech is affected and there is tightening of the closing muscles. Because the vertical dimension of occlusion is determined by the contracted length of the powerful closing muscles, any violation of that position by increasing space can begin the physiological process of increasing muscle activity, returning to the original vertical.

Once any amount of restorative prosthodontic or implant dentistry is placed, it is certainly possible for muscle response to be in apposition of closing muscle activity. Therefore, it is strongly suggested that whenever vertical opening is planned, the clinician should evaluate the amount of free-way space by measuring the difference between closed contact and rest position. A dot placed on the chin and a dot placed on the nose are easy reference points. Measure that distance with the patient closed, and then measure the rest dimension by saying "Emma" and holding on the "M" sound. This can be repeated several times until a consistent rest dimension is recorded.

The difference between the rest and closed dimensions is the free-way space, which should never be violated by opening past that number. A good rule to remember is that some room can be stolen from the free-way space but never taken away completely. That violation makes any future dentistry very difficult, as often that violated patient becomes an occlusal neurotic. These patients tend to want their occlusion changed often, and for unknown reasons want their bite opened more. In most cases, it is best to leave the patient at the original vertical, even if equilibration is desired.

If vertical needs to be opened for prosthetic convenience, a little room should be taken from the existing free-way space. If the patient has very little free-way space, then opening should not be contemplated. Ask the patient to count aloud from one to ten. If the teeth hit before six or seven, there is very little free-way space and opening should not be contemplated.

In the case of true bite collapse, lost vertical can be restored and this is not considered opening the vertical dimension of occlusion. In the case of lost vertical, the vertical restoration provides greater freedom for speech and crown-to-root ratio when opening past the rest position.

Step 2B: Set The Incisal Pin

This is an important and routine step. The vertical dimension is recorded by unlocking the centric lock, lifting the incisal pin off of the table, and

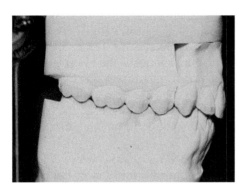
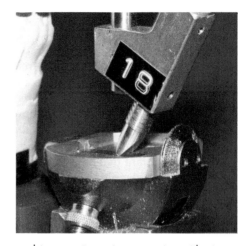

Figs. 10.4 and 10.5. Casts squeezed into maximum intercuspation with pin on table.

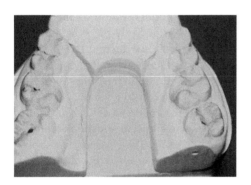
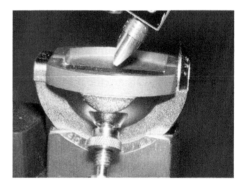

Figs. 10.6 and 10.7. Casts marking first point of contact with open pin.

squeezing and sliding the articulated casts into maximum intercuspation (figs. 10.4 and 10.5). Once the pin is dropped onto the table and locked into place, the vertical dimension of occlusion at the acquired bite is recorded. At this point, the clinician should separate the casts and lock the case back into centric relation arc of closure, first point of contact (figs. 10.6). At this time, the clinician may notice there is a pin that is off the table (fig. 10.7).

Again, the more open the vertical dimension is, the easier the equilibration will be. If it doesn't open much, it is important to be cautious and attempt to close the cast through trial equilibration techniques. The accuracy of the centric relation record is critical from this step forward. This author typically uses bite splint therapy prior to making the CR record, in order to improve accuracy. Even a slightly misdiagnosed set of articulated casts can lead to an inappropriate treatment plan. If CR is missed, then all the steps can lead to erroneous treatment.

Step 3A: Work Out Edge-to-Edge and Crossover Details along with Mandibular Incisal Plane

A major indication of the maturity and experience level of the clinician is the willingness to adjust or alter the mandibular incisal edge of a patient going through an occlusal reorganization. As has already been pointed out, one cannot get precise, appropriate edge match-ups if the lower plane is not corrected to a horizontally level, even, and smooth working blade. This level of maturity is reached earlier by the ability to correct an opposing quadrant that has supererupted and the willingness to talk to the patient about the pitfalls of leaving an uneven plane of occlusion and an uneven lower incisal plane.

Figures 10.8 through 10.10 demonstrate how we can use crossover information to establish the appropriate and dominant position of the upper incisal edge.

If there is any interest or concern about the esthetics of the anterior teeth or the patient is questioning smile appearance, the author recommends investigating the edges of all anterior teeth early on in the diagnostic process. The same holds true during the trial equilibration or the actual clinical additive and/or subtractive adjustment. A likely place to start the esthetic examination is the upper smile analysis, conducting the analysis as one would to set denture teeth in a wax rim. Important elements of the analysis are the midline, buccal corridor, esthetic smile line, incisal length, gingival height, and phonetic correctness of the incisal edges.

The esthetic expectations of patients and the ability to deliver naturally beautiful fixed restorations have increased the clinician's responsibility to understand the fundamentals of a patient's smile. The clinician also must predictably accomplish fixed improvements to the smile without violating both the envelope of function and the envelope of parafunction. The following chart indicates a time-proven analysis that has worked for this author for many years.

Step-by-Step Analysis of Mandibular Incisal Edge

1. Observe and photograph lips at repose.
2. Observe and photograph full (big) smile.
3. Evaluate the length-to-width ratio of the teeth.
4. Evaluate the gingival display.
5. Evaluate and photograph left and right crossover contact positions.
6. Evaluate and photograph the protrusive contact position.
7. Evaluate the lips while the patient makes "F" and "S" sounds.
8. Evaluate the lip closure path.
9. Observe the midline, incisal plane, and buccal corridor.

Many of these steps will be familiar from the full denture protocol. Two additions are evaluating the protrusive and crossover contact positions

Parafunctional Cross-Over

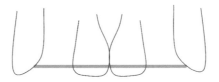

Lower Incisal Plane

Switching from Cuspids to Centrals

Parafunctional Cross-Over

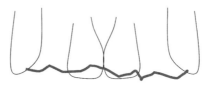

Lower Incisal Plane

**Requires Level Lower Incisal Plane
or It Cannot Function Smoothly**

Parafunctional Cross-Over

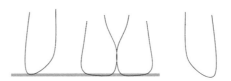

Lower Incisal Plane

**Smooth – Going Out and Coming Back
Needs the Dominance of the Central Incisors**

Figs. 10.8–10.10. Using crossover information to establish appropriate upper incisal edge.

(steps 5 and 6) Once the clinician gets crossover adjusted properly, the protrusive edge-to-edge contact of the centrals is even or can be quickly adjusted because the edge-to-edge position of the centrals in both protrusive and crossover is the same. The reader can easily observe this phenomenon by carefully adjusting a lower bite splint into a smooth crossover and then observing that, by going into protrusive, the edge-to-edge positions will be just about perfectly even (figs. 10.11 through 10.18).

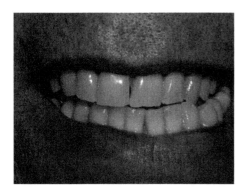 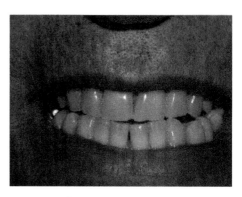

Figs. 10.11 and 10.12. Irregular improper edges.

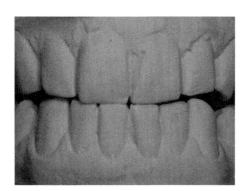 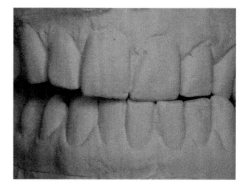

Figs. 10.13 and 10.14. Corrected casts.

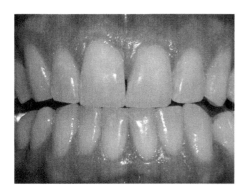 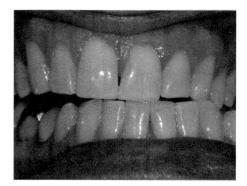

Figs. 10.15 and 10.16. Corrected teeth.

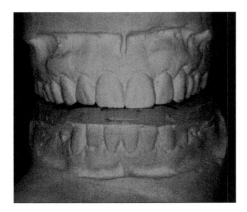
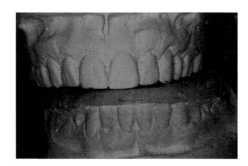

Figs. 10.17 and 10.18. Corrected occlusal bite splint.

The question remains how long the two maxillary centrals should or could be. From a functional point of view they should be dominant so that they can take the hand off of the lower incisal plane as it begins to cross over past the cuspid cusp tips.

At the start of the diagnostic workup, it is sensible to begin with planning to correct the lower incisal plane, if it needs to be corrected, so the crossover will be smooth. This will eventually be accomplished by either shortening the tall irregular teeth or building up the short irregular teeth, but it is premature to decide whether orthodontics, adjustment, and/or restorative means will be the most appropriate.

The clinician may look at the upper cuspids and their relationship to the existing bicuspids and the rest of the smile line. It could be that all teeth involved need correcting or just the cuspids. The following list offers suggestions as to how to approach the details of these changes.

Steps for Creating a Level and Esthetic Plane of Occlusion

1. Work with the cuspid-to-central-length ratio. The centrals must be dominant.
2. Make sure the lower cuspid is within the mandibular incisal plane.
3. Work out the details of incisal edges.
4. Bevel the labial maxillary cuspid edge.
5. Bevel the lingual mandibular cuspid edge.
6. Redo all the incisal embrasures.

Note that almost every time a lower cuspid is left sticking up above the rest of the plane of occlusion, it serves as an interference. Often this heightened canine crashes into the upper lateral in protrusive movement. This explains the need for an increased incisal embrasure between upper lateral and upper cuspids. None of the other often-stated rules of esthetics give the clinician a specific way to determine the length of the maxillary central incisors.

Some clinicians like to use the big "E" smile, some the lips at rest, some the normal length-to-width ratio, and some the average length. It seems to this author that these are all helpful but not definitive. When the crossover is made just right, the adjustment seems to produce the most esthetic length of upper centrals. This length seems to be the most normal appearing in ratio with the length of the other anterior teeth. And the best news is that this length of the upper centrals has the best chance to hold up for a long time, even in the presence of parafunctional habits. This observation goes a long way in illustrating the ultimate and undeniable relationship between function and esthetics or, more simply stated, between form and function.

The other big question remains as to what to do with the lower incisal plane. Should it be lowered or raised to make it level, horizontal, and smooth? In truth, it is often simply clinical judgment. However, there are penalties to pay in the case of certain choices.

1. When the plane is lowered, there is a tendency for this to increase the need for posterior equilibration so the amount and quality of enamel left on the remaining teeth could influence the clinician's decision.
2. On the other hand, when the incisal plane is raised, it is not uncommon to then need to increase vertical dimension so the contours of the upper anterior teeth won't have to be significantly ground away in severe violation of basic anterior guidance principles. The amount of free-way space, a history of muscle hyperactivity, and/or joint dysfunction would counterindicate increasing the vertical dimension. The one most-often cited reason for increasing vertical dimension is for prosthetic convenience when the case requires extensive restorations and there is not enough room to place the restorations.

If the patient has sufficient free-way space, the clinician should not hesitate to test out the new vertical in provisionals or bonded composite interim mocked-up restorations (figs. 10.19–10.22). A critical part of this testing is to evaluate the ease and clarity of phonetics, and to note whether posterior teeth hit prior to the patient's counting aloud to six or seven.

When modifying the lower incisal plane, remember to recreate natural and youthful appearing incisal embrasures. If this is not accomplished, leveling the plane will greatly age the appearance of the smile. Small diamond discs can be used to recreate the arrowhead appearance of natural embrasures. The recreation will allow the patient to slide floss into interproximal spaces. Obviously, as in all other adjustments, a fine, polished finish must be obtained.

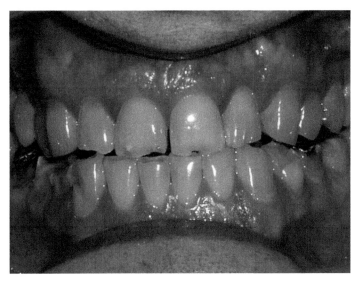

Fig. 10.19. Pre-operative photo of bonded case demonstrating the option of opening vertical dimension. Courtesy of Dr. Daren Becker.

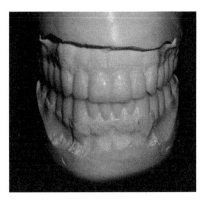

Fig. 10.20. Diagnostic workup of above case. Courtesy of Matt Roberts, CDT.

Often the clinician can Pindex the posterior quadrants of one or the other casts so that the anterior edge work can be accomplished free of posterior interferences. This little diversion allows the astute clinician to preview the potential anterior guidance and whether the anterior contacts will fall into a reasonable relationship after posterior equilibration. It will also help the clinician to determine whether orthodontics or greater restorative techniques will be required to achieve anterior coupling. Thus, a lot can be answered without the need of time-consuming posterior equilibration (figs. 10.23–10.27).

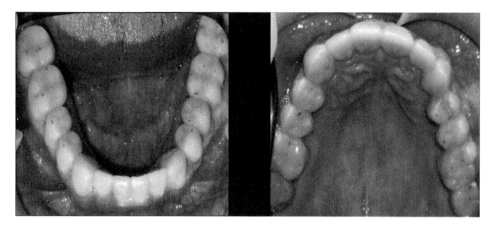

Fig. 10.21. Adjusted occlusion on composite. Mock-up of above case. Courtesy of Dr. Daren Becker.

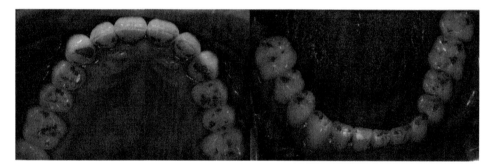

Fig. 10.22. Five-year follow-up of feldspathic porcelain over lava core. Finished occlusion of complex case with increased vertical dimension of occlusion. Courtesy of Dr. Daren Becker.

Step 3B: Reshape and Warp Posterior Cusps, Fossa, and Inclines

Although equilibration of posterior teeth is complex, most clinicians can expect to gain confidence by trial equilibrating 10 to 15 different cases.

One way to look at posterior tooth equilibration is to imagine Michelangelo removing stone that is in the wrong places. The approach of grinding away occlusal marks that appear to be in inappropriate places implies one knows where the marks actually should be. A healthy occlusal contact is made up of a cusp tip and an opposing landing area. Thus, occlusal marks actually should be on any existing or created small flat landing area called a "centrum." These landing areas should be in

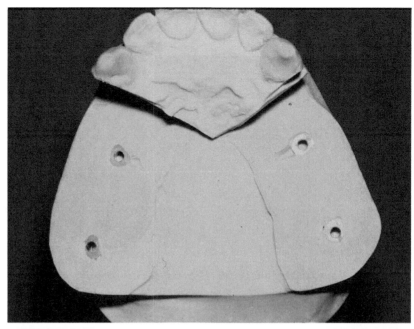

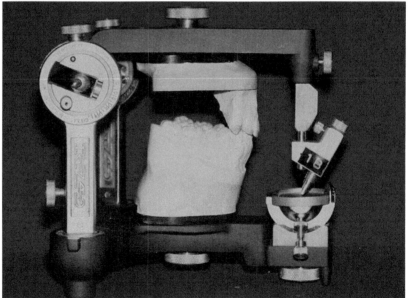

Figs. 10.23 and 10.24. Evaluating coupling possibility on Pindexed model.

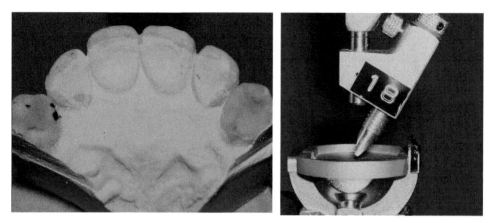

Figs. 10.25 and 10.26. Note first point of anterior contact with open pin.

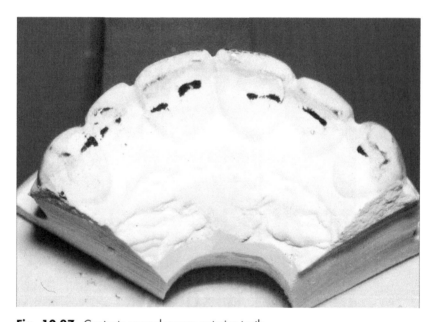

Fig. 10.27. Contacts spread across anterior teeth.

the center, bucco-lingually, of each posterior tooth, and thus not on an incline.

Contacts should not be on inclines away from the idealized central receiving areas, as contacts on inclines can be detrimental to tooth structure and muscle activity and can possibly affect the susceptibility of periodontal disease. Incline contacts can be the precursor of shifts in mandibular

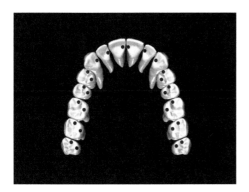 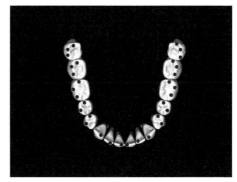

Figs. 10.28 and 10.29. Idealized locations of centric stops. Both figures © 2010 Wolters Kluwer Health/Lippincott Williams and Wilkins. Reprinted with permission.

closure, leading to increased muscle activity. These interferences can be the microtrauma that leads to tissue degradation in the temporomandibular joint.

Figures 10.28 and 10.29 demonstrate an ideal set of marks from a Class I perspective. Note that contacts on the mandibular teeth are often near the distal marginal ridge or fossa area and that contacts on the maxillary teeth are often near the mesial marginal ridges or fossa area. If a well-formed and rounded opposing cusp exists, the mark is on or near the cusp tip.

Another way to think about posterior tooth equilibration is to think of the process as if it were related to orthodontics. One could think of the need to warp a given cusp to a better position since, in the centric relation arc of closure, it is hitting on an incline contact. One could grind, shape, or warp the offending cusp tip area in the precise same direction as one would want the receiving mark to move toward a better-defined centrum (fig. 10.30). The requisite hand-eye coordination is precisely why dentists need to pass the spatial relationship part of the dental aptitude test upon entering dental school.

Picture an imaginary string connecting the cusp tip and the receiving area. To move the receiving area in a given direction, the cusp tip needs to be warped in the same direction. The only problem is that the clinician is looking at all of this upside down and usually in the mirror.

As grinding begins, usually with either a small diamond wheel bur or a diamond football-shaped bur, the receiving mark is expected to move slightly with each subsequent marking. At one point, the next mark will show no contact. This can be frustrating unless the operator remembers that now some other first point of contact is hitting on another tooth. The grinding process is then begun on the next tooth that begins to hit. This process is repeated over many teeth until all marks are hitting in more preferred places.

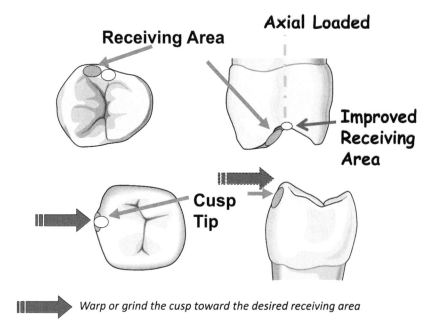

Receiving Area

Axial Loaded

Improved Receiving Area

Cusp Tip

Warp or grind the cusp toward the desired receiving area

Fig. 10.30. Warping of cusp tips to improve position of receiving areas.

Equilibration Involves Three Basic Steps

1. **Read the receiving area.** This means that before any grinding is begun, the clinician observes the particular receiving area and decides in which direction it would be best to move it. This observation is made on the receiving area, as the cusp tip mark may not be as instructive. It must be remembered that adjustment can be done on and around the cusp tip area in the attempt to improve the location of the landing area. The clinician should keep in mind that as the patient is guided into the centric relation arc of closure and the first point of contact begins to hit, the mandible will open compared to its maximum inter-cuspation. Grinding can be done as long as the case is still at an open vertical. The goal is minimal tooth reduction that gets the dots lined up just as an orthodontist would align cusp tips.
2. **Warp, shape, and grind the offensive cusp tip area.** This step is the actual removal of tooth structure to eliminate incline contact and to effectively move the receiving area toward the long axis position. If a cusp tip interference is the major problem, then it is addressed first. Once in a while, the excursive interferences are the major part of the problem, and then they are addressed first. If the trial equilibration is skipped, then the operator could either go too far or not take enough away, thus inadvertently changing the vertical dimension of occlusion.

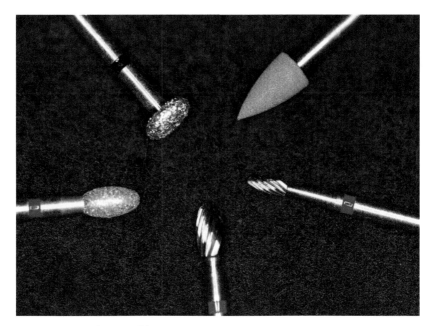

Fig. 10.31. Selection of burs.

A trial equilibration on casts leads to a clear vision of where to start and where to end, and this clear vision is important when making irreversible change. Coarse diamonds are used in the beginning, and then fine diamonds and eventually carbide finishing burs are utilized. This author always ends with polishing points so that the teeth appear not to have been ground (figs. 10.31 and 10.32).

3. **Go back and erase the old incline mark at or surrounding the errone-ous centrum.** This adjustment accomplishes two things. One, it helps the excursive movement out of centric. (This will be described in greater detail later.) Two, it eliminates the need to do all of the adjustment around the cusp tip area. Any steep inclines that could serve as excur-sive interferences are thus leveled off during the centric adjustment.

Many of this author's students have had difficulty with these three steps because they remember being told that one never grinds the centric holding cusp tip. That is correct when the patient is at the desired final vertical dimension of occlusion.

Please remember that when a trial equilibration or the actual equilibra-tion is started intraorally, it is almost always starting at an increased verti-cal. Therefore, it is permissible to reduce the centric holding cusp tip while still in the open situation. Once final vertical dimension of occlusion is achieved, then the holding cusp tip should not be touched. This is precisely why two different color-marking papers are used—to always identify the final centric marks while adjusting excursive interferences.

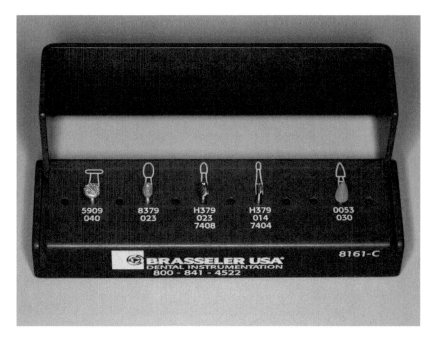

Fig. 10.32. Equilibration bur kit.

Removing a precious centric-holding cusp tip could be a disaster after working hard to achieve it in the final vertical dimension of occlusion position. A good rule to follow is to use black for centric and red for excursive markings so black can be laid over the red excursive markings.

Step 4: Return to Original Vertical or Planned Vertical

In keeping with equilibrating according to an orthodontic mindset (leveling and aligning), this step is similar to the leveling objective of many orthodontic protocols. In the previous steps, aligning was the objective. Assuming the clinician has achieved adequate alignment and the case is still open, the clinician no longer needs to align the receiving areas by warping cusp position. If some or many cusps are still hitting high, the clinician now has to decide which surface to reduce—the cusp tip area or the fossa landing area.

If a given tooth is still high and its cusp tip is longer than the rest of the plane of occlusion, the cusp tip should be shortened. Analyzing the given plane of occlusion prior to beginning the adjustment is prudent. Observing the smile line helps in deciding where to reduce. If the maxillary cuspid is in an appropriate smile line but its adjacent bicuspid is too long for a pleasant appearance, then the bicuspid should be reduced. If the bicuspid looks good, then the opposing lower cuspid receiving area should be reduced. The concept of form and function going hand in hand again holds true.

If the plane of occlusion and smile line are not a consideration, one can attempt to not deepen the receiving area in order to make it much more difficult for posterior disclusion. The one exception is when there is an overabundance of steepness coming from the anterior guidance or condylar inclination. In this case, a much steeper cusp-fossa inclination can be utilized.

Every dentist has a favorite or more comfortable quadrant in which to work. One must resist the temptation to make all adjustments in one quadrant or risk taking too much off of one area and inadvertently destroying precious enamel and/or an existing restoration that does not need to be replaced. Adjustments should be spread across all quadrants, and demolition of healthy tooth structure and existing restorations should be avoided. When finished, the equilibrated mouth should have enhanced anatomical features and an improved smile (figs. 10.33–10.35).

Step 5: Remove All Balancing and Protrusive Interferences

There is not much to think about when deciding whether to remove balancing and/or protrusive interferences. The balancing and protrusive marks need to be removed with aggressiveness. The other excursive marks may need some thought, especially if it is not an easy case to obtain cuspid guidance.

Whenever marking balancing interferences, the patient should be instructed to move with power from outside in. Have the patient do a practice move out to cuspid cusp tip and crunch back to home base prior to placing the marking media. Coach the patient to mimic the parafunctional forces they make when grinding back to closure. The point being that if a patient only moves from cuspid to closure without power, the balancing side contacts probably will not be detrimental.

Practice also should be accomplished prior to protrusive marking. Have the patient start out at the edge-to-edge position and then crunch back to closure, sliding on the lingual surfaces of the anterior maxillary teeth. It is only during simulation of parafunction that the clinician observes the full effect of closing muscles really firing up during the glide back to closure.

Almost all muscle studies indicate there is parafunctional hyperactivity of the powerful closing muscles precisely when excursive interferences are grinding over each other. These powerful muscles actually get the balancing side condyles to seat further during their trip back home. Also, the mandible can bend ever so slightly during the parafunctional movement, exhibiting powerful muscle firing.

When the patient moves from closure onto the cuspid or other guiding teeth, not as much force is delivered. Before grinding, remember to mark

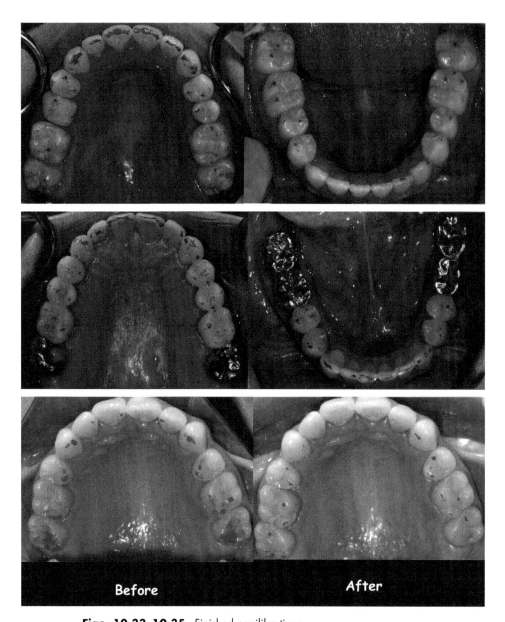

Figs. 10.33–10.35. Finished equilibrations.

the centric contacts in black and to mark the balancing or any other excursive contacts in red.

It has been this author's finding that one of the most destructive interferences can be on the third molars during protrusive movement. Note a worn incline on the third molar during protrusive that may mimic the condylar incline. This apparently occurs because the third molars are so far back toward the joint apparatus and receive the brunt of the lever system effect. The interference is directly alongside of the powerful closing muscle. Check to see if the condylar inclination is dialed in close to the actual inclination. If there is a discrepancy between third molar wear inclines in protrusive and the condylar setting, this could be a red flag pointing out an error.

Be aware that sometimes the interference is not simply tooth structure. It is possible to have soft tissue serve as an interference, for example, the retromolar pad during protrusive movement. Sometimes it is the posterior tuberosity. Occasionally the only corrective solution is surgery.

Step 6: Cuspid Guidance—Unless a Compromise Is Required

Even though a separate chapter is dedicated to anterior guidance, this step deserves its own number. Numerous debates and articles have been written about the benefits of cuspid guidance. Because the cusp has the longest root and the best corner position, this author sees no reason to allow other teeth to take the immediate load of guiding the mandible out of centric when the cusp is in a proper position to be coupled. The cuspid is the cornerstone of the maxilla and demonstrates no evidence of pathology when asked to do guidance, other than in parafunctional destructive situations.

Optimal guidance occurs when the gliding of the lower cusp tip is along the mesial half of the upper cuspid. Thus, no distalizing effect can occur unless the lower cusp tip is tracking down the distal slope of the upper cuspid. This distal tracking could become a detrimental influence on the working side condyle disc assembly, especially if there is some degree of parafunctional activity present. Unfortunately, this is found occasionally in the Class II situation, simply because of the retrognathic effect.

If the cusp can't be coupled because of arch size discrepancy, Class II–Division I occlusal relationships, periodontal conditions (cuspid too weak to guide), or because it is simply missing or out of position, compromise may be necessary leading to a form of group function or involving one or both bicuspids until the cuspid can take over. When compromise is needed, care must be taken to create a minimal initial guidance stroke on the bicuspid and a very smooth transition to the cuspid as soon as possible. Some clinicians have called this a "progressive guidance forward." This author feels strongly that this compromise should be utilized only when cuspid contact in centric is impossible.

One warning is to never build out a form on either cuspid, which is not naturally found in nature, just to make contact with the opposing cuspid. When this type of overcontouring is attempted, the periodontal condition is usually compromised, occlusal stability is lessoned, the tongue has to accommodate in a bothersome manner, and/or phonetics is negatively affected.

When coupling is not possible, the decision needs to be made whether to treat orthodontically or even surgically. Clear, consistent communication with the patient about the consequences of not treating the condition can lead to an educated decision made mutually by both patient and clinician. The consequences of not treating the condition are continued muscle activity, tooth wear and breakage, loss of stability, tooth mobility and migration, and even food impaction due to loss of good interproximal contact. Both parties must be aware of these possibilities when guidance is left on bicuspids. However, sometimes there are no alternatives if other treatment choices are either refused or inappropriate.

Another consideration is whether the patient has perfectly adapted to group function. Signs of perfect adaptation are the absence of wear, mobility, and muscle tenderness.

The correct or appropriate style guidance may be tested in detail during the patient's bite splint therapy. If there is a question about which direction to take, the group function can be first attempted on the bite splint and the result evaluated.

Previously cited clinical studies have demonstrated that patients better accept the reduction of anterior guidance incline steepness and that there is reduced muscle activity when guidance is moved more forward. But if there is no apparent ill affect from the current guidance, why not leave it as is? Figures 10.36 through 10.41 demonstrate various guidance styles chosen for each individual case.

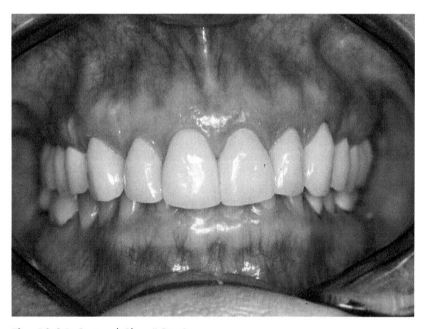

Fig. 10.36. Restored Class II Div 2.

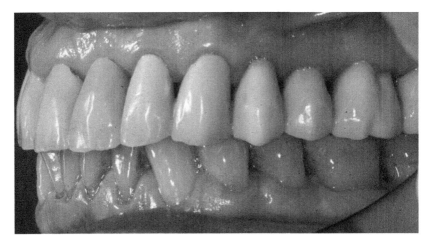

Fig. 10.37. Class I restored with acrylic provisionals. Courtesy of Dr. Irwin Becker.

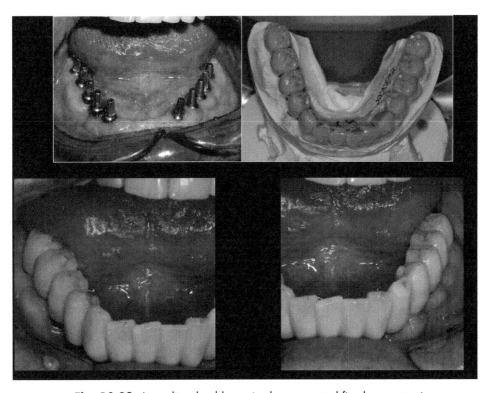

Fig. 10.38. Immediate load lower implant supported fixed reconstruction.

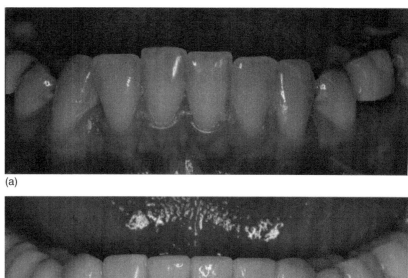

(a)

(b)

Fig. 10.39. a. Pre-op. b. Restored Class II Div 2.

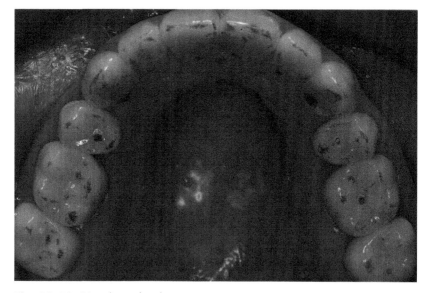

Fig. 10.40. Note lingualized centric stops.

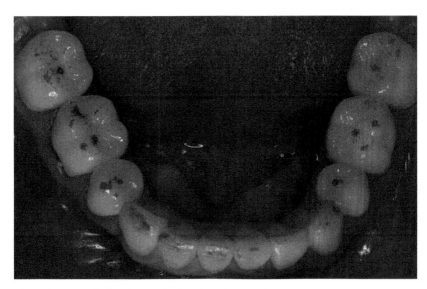

Fig. 10.41. Labialized incisal labial bevel centric stops.

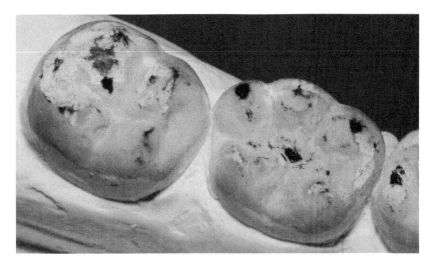

Fig. 10.42. Choices of centric stops: (1) Create groove distal to disto-buccal cusp. (2) Sacrifice disto-buccal cusp. (3) Sacrifice central pit receiving area.

One of the most perplexing puzzles is how to get all or most centric cusp tips to make stable contact on opposing teeth. Figure 10.42 illustrates when an upper centric cusp tip travels directly over a lower centric holding cusp tip. There is a dilemma deciding which centric stop to sacrifice. During the trial equilibration, the clinician may learn how to warp one or both so they will not eventually bump into to each other, but sometimes this is inevitable.

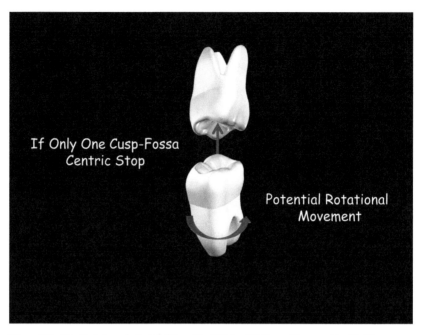

Fig. 10.43. Rotational instability. © 2010 Wolters Kluwer Health/Lippincott Williams and Wilkins. Reprinted with permission.

It seems to make the most sense to make sure at least one upper and one lower centric holding cusp tip are touching. If one cusp tip is sacrificed, let it be the one that leaves another of its adjacent cusps in contact. An example is if both lower buccal cusps are touching in centric but the distal buccal cusp is interfering with the sole upper lingual cusp. If the distal buccal of the lower were to be sacrificed, it would leave one lower buccal and one upper lingual in centric contact (fig. 10.42). This author pictures these contacts as a stapling effect, especially if a stable interproximal contact exists, as the two teeth will not move and be in a stable situation. When only one cusp contacts in centric, it is possible for one tooth to rotate around the one cusp tip. Figure 10.43 demonstrates rotational instability.

Step 7: Work Out Anterior Guidance

There is no one exact way to describe how to customize anterior guidance for each case. Optimally, the appropriate set of teeth that are the most forward will do the guidance and they will be made up of the shallowest inclines that still disclude the rest of the posterior teeth. Remember that the appropriate guidance also has to look attractive and function well with phonetic requirements. Optimal guidance generally runs down the marginal ridges of the upper anterior teeth; however, the precise placement depends on the position, alignment, and periodontal condition of these teeth.

Commonly used diagrams show the upper two central incisors guiding in protrusive. This guidance is satisfactory if the central incisors are strong. If the central incisors have deeper pockets and demonstrate some increasing mobility, then the guidance will be more appropriately spread across four or more anterior teeth.

If the lower anterior teeth are poorly aligned, then the guidance will not be well placed on marginal ridges of the upper central incisors. During equilibration procedures, the clinician may be able to reshape the lower anterior teeth slightly so that any parts of the lower incisors that are protrusive relative to arch form alignment may be made to appear in better alignment, thus helping to get the guidance more appropriately placed on marginal ridges (figs. 10.44 and 10.45). As natural contours are regained, often a better functional guidance is achieved.

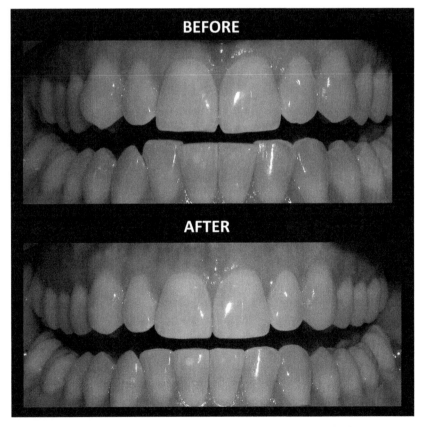

Figs. 10.44 and 10.45. Improving alignment through shaping of edges to accomplish optimal guidance.

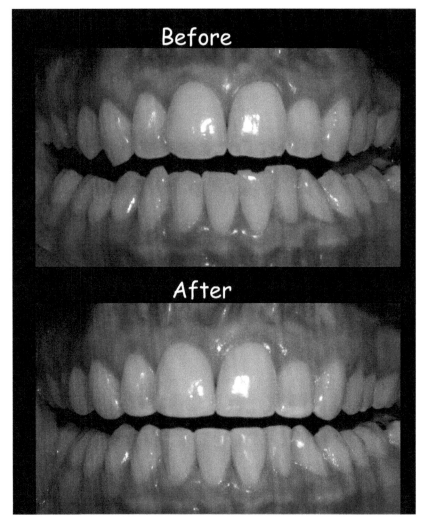

Figs. 10.44 and 10.45. *Continued*

When attempting to adjust centric stops on upper anterior teeth, it is important not to grind a hole or depression out of which the lower incisal edge will have great difficulty gliding (figs. 10.46–10.49). A planing motion is desired. Reduce the high spot, keeping the natural contour in mind. This adjustment is enhanced by remembering to split the adjustment between both the flat top of the lower incisor, called the "pitch," and the leading labial incisal line angle, which most often contains the centric mark. Also on this angle is the bevel that does the gliding out of centric and onto the marginal ridges for guidance. So in reality there are three distinct places to adjust: (a) receiving area on upper anterior tooth, (b) pitch of the flat incisal edge, and (c) the bevel made up of the labial incisal angle.

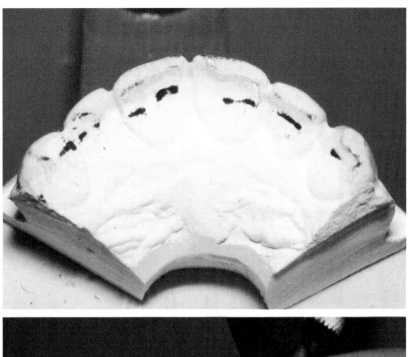

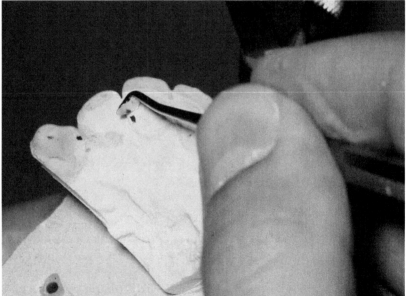

Figs. 10.46–10.49. The technique of adjusting anterior guidance: (1) Level lower anteriors. (2) Warp lower cuspids and bicuspids. (3) Don't dig hole for CR stops. (4) Maintain cuspid angle until posterior teeth are replaced.

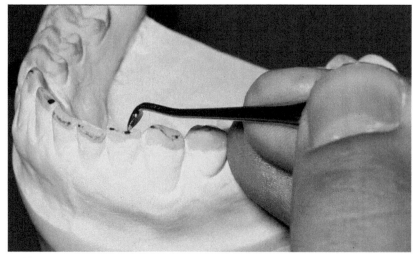

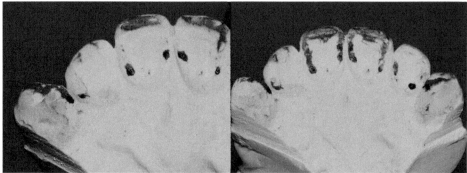

Figs. 10.46–10.49. *Continued*

The same delicate adjustment that is used to work out the anterior edge of the mandibular bite splint is applied in this procedure. Often this adjustment is smoothed by sandpaper discs, rubber wheels, and points. It is a delicate adjustment, achieving a light centric contact and very smooth imperceptible movement from one edge to the other. Ask the patient if he or she can feel when one tooth touches and the other takes over. Optimally, the patient cannot answer that question. During the trial equilibration, learn to hold onto the condylar housing and move on the edges and crossover positions to feel any catch or bump (fig. 10.50). The clinician should not be able to tell when the teeth are actually touching.

While equilibrating the guidance and then evaluating the working (inner) inclines of the upper buccal cusps, the operator should picture steepness decreasing from cuspid angle to molar incline. Practice holding the diamond wheel bur to reflect that change from anterior to posterior. Figure 10.51 demonstrates this technique. This will create condylar guid-

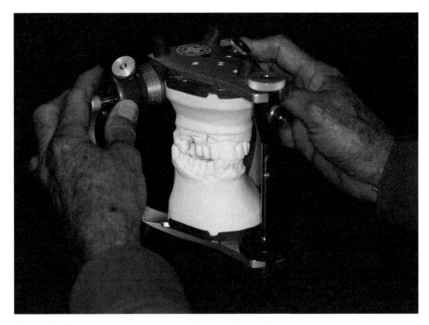

Fig. 10.50. How to move the articulator while feeling every catch.

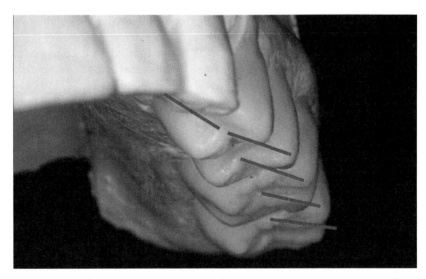

Fig. 10.51. The reduction in steepness of working inclines from cuspid to molar.

ance that has greater influence posteriorly than anteriorly, and also increased separation between the posterior inclines, which is desired because of potential mandibular flexing.

Step 8: Evaluate Curve of Wilson

This step is one of both observation and occasional adjustment. When this step is overlooked, and it commonly is, the patient may present with a sore or painful tooth and no apparent explanation. This is because the patient cannot explain or describe when it actually hurts unless the patient moves over into a distinct parafunctional position and crunches on the incline interference way over in parafunction. This typically occurs when a loser lingual cusp tip is unnaturally high and interferes with the upper buccal cusp tip of its opponent tooth.

This violation of Curve of Wilson can be observed even before the patient moves into excursion (fig. 10.52). Almost every time there is an exaggerated violation of this curve, the possibility of excursive interference exists. It seems as if the lingual cusps of lower molars serve the sole purpose of holding food on the molars' table-like surfaces. As mentioned in other chapters, it is not known exactly why a patient would move over into the bizarre parafunctional position, but the clinician has the responsibility to not leave tooth structure or restorative material in a position that could become an interference.

Thus, there are two areas of concern when it comes to adjusting for parafunction—both the anterior aspect that leads to a smooth gliding effect and the posterior drag that could simulate the same kind of negative consequences as balancing posterior interferences. When these posterior types of interferences occur on the balancing side, they not only harm tooth

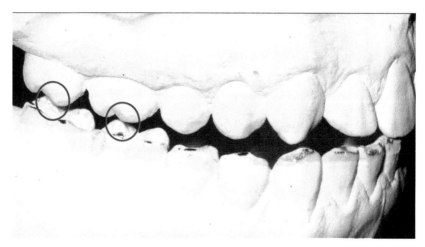

Fig. 10.52. Curve of Wilson violation: interferences of lower lingual cusps during parafunction.

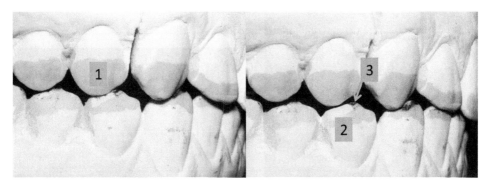

Fig. 10.53. Choices based on esthetic smile line (excursive adjustment choices): (1) If upper bicuspid is long, then shorten it. (2) If upper bicuspid is correct, then shorten lower cusp. (3) The one place not to adjust is the centric stop.

structure and muscle but also can stimulate a process of tissue degradation from the production of cytokines. The microtrauma that occurs on the top of the interfering teeth transfers up the mandibular ramus and into the condyle disc assembly.

This author routinely recontours these specific inclines even if they are not symptomatic. This adjustment seems to also help out mastication by improving the food table.

Be aware that an interference can occur when the upper buccal cusp is hanging down so markedly that it rubs against the lower lingual cusp. From an esthetic evaluation, the clinician should be able to pick up the upper cusp that is obtrusive to the smile line (fig. 10.53). This observation demonstrates once again that better function leads to better esthetics and vice versa.

Step 9: Allow for Freedom in Centric

This step involves an understanding of tooth morphology and the evolution of occlusal understanding. Historically, there have been two accepted approaches to shaping occlusal contacts. The tripod approach attempts to achieve the natural, unworn, and pristine occlusal contact of a young adult. The tripod approach reached its prominent usage during the active use of gnathological principles. The cusp-to-fossa approach is a more therapeutic style.

The tripod style requires a detailed understanding of the stomatognathic system. It requires the use of a fully adjustable articulator in order to achieve immediate posterior disclusion. The fully adjustable articulator can more accurately provide the specific pathways and sluiceways for cusps to pass out of their tripoded centric stops.

The cusp-to-fossa style requires basic knowledge of anatomy and a basic articulator that can accept an approximate facebow instead of the more

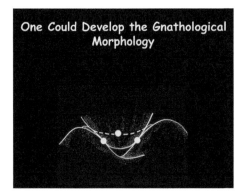
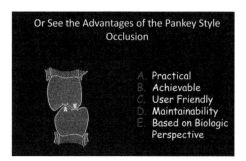

Figs. 10.54 and 10.55. Benefits of flat receiving area.

accurate hinge axis locator. This is because it is much easier to disclude when the nicely formed rounded cusp tip exits off of a centrum. Basic knowledge of ridge and groove direction allows for this kind of disclusion on almost all types of restorative cases and the trial equilibration during case workup. One gets used to this style by adjusting lots of flat plane bite splints.

Another benefit of the cusp-to-fossa style is that it seems to be more stable over the long term. If any changes occur in tooth or condyle position after morphology is tripoded, multiple incline contacts will be immediately noticed and be accompanied by the return of negative sequelae. However, if any changes occur on cusp-to-fossa contacts, there are almost no negative consequences. Figures 10.54 and 10.55 demonstrate why this author prefers the cusp-to-fossa morphology with flat receiving areas.

It is also very important to remember that freedom in centric requires the clinician to check the equilibration after establishing the maximum number of centric stops. The decision may be made to allow anterior teeth less firm contact in comparison with posterior contacts.

Have the patient sit upright and tilt his or her head slightly forward when evaluating anterior contacts. Not only ask how these anterior teeth feel, but also place your fingers over the six anterior teeth while the patient is tapping. If any fremitus is felt, then continue with slight reduction using a rubber (composite) point. Remember, these teeth should not be taken out of occlusion, just left touching lighter. The visiting faculty at the Pankey Institute are frequently surveyed and continually report their patients feel better with this style of finishing.

Step 10: Refine Centric Stops to a Halo

An often-overlooked fact, when attempting to read the marks from any sort of marking ribbon or marking paper, is that the size of the mark has nothing to do with how hard the contact is hitting. The size of the mark is related to the size and shape of the opposing cusp tip. A large, flat cusp tip will create a large, broad mark. Do not mistake this mark as the hardest hitting spot. A sharp-pointed cusp may leave a tiny mark, but it could be the cusp that is hitting the hardest.

So, how does the clinician know which mark is hitting hardest and should be the mark to begin adjusting? Utilize the marking ribbon to carry the ink onto the receiving area, then immediately tap on the same spot with the ribbon in place. Look carefully with magnifiers to see which mark or marks have a slightly clear center. The clear center is where teeth are hitting the hardest and the cusp tip is wiping off a bit of the ink.

The hardest contacts with clear centers are the ones that should be adjusted first. The marks should be taken away to the thickness of the ink. The thickness of the ribbon is not important. The ultimate goal is to have all of the marks hitting at the same time, with each having a hole in the center. These holes have been variously called the "halo," "doughnut," "bull's eye," or "bagel." Anterior contacts might not have as clear a center as the posterior contacts.

Please review carefully the examples shown in figures 10.56 and 10.57 that demonstrate how accurate the clinician can be. Riise (1982) demonstrated how accurate the clinician must be to predictably turn off excessive muscle activity. The reported 30- to 50-micron dimension can be achieved by using polishing points and adjusting to the thickness of the ink.

This author occasionally attempts an alternative technique to help guide a patient during equilibration procedures, namely, an internal deprogrammer (fig. 10.58). The deprogrammer is created by bonding in a small amount of composite to the lingual of the maxillary central incisors. As the internal deprogrammer is adjusted, the first point of contact soon appears.

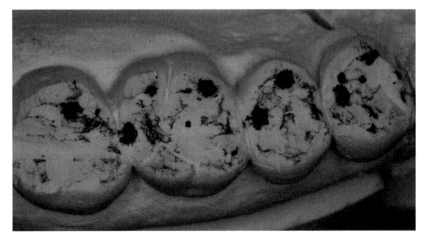

Fig. 10.56. Tap with ribbon in place.

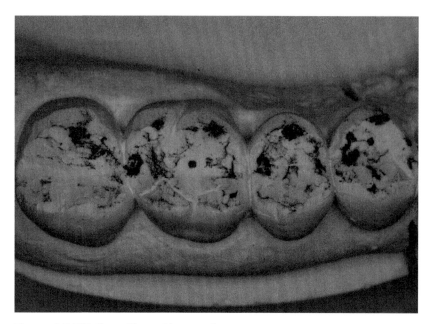

Figure 10.57. Tap without ribbon in place.

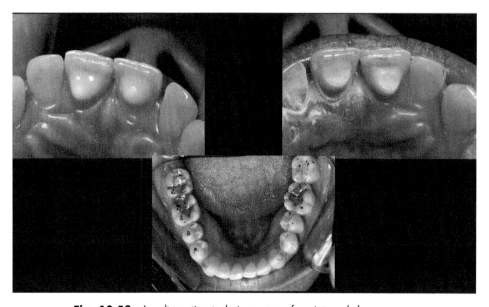

Fig. 10.58. An alternative technique: use of an internal deprogrammer.

Then both tooth structure and deprogrammer are adjusted. Eventually, there is no more deprogrammer left to adjust, at which time the original vertical dimension is achieved. Rarely is it difficult to guide a patient into centric relation arc of closure after bite splint therapy has been attempted. This technique is utilized for these difficult patients but not if there are severe joint conditions.

SUMMARY OF THE TEN STEPS OF EQUILIBRATION

The previously described steps present the details needed to understand both the actual equilibration and the trial equilibration. The following summary will serve as an easy reference, allowing the clinician to think through and achieve any case that is mounted in centric relation arc of closure. Follow the steps and the pictures while doing any trial equilibration. Trial equilibrations are easiest when there is some amount of vertical opening at the first point of contact. For your first case, select one that needs posterior restoration, so that any error in equilibration can be corrected during tooth preparation.

1. Evaluate anterior guidance in habitual occlusion.
2. Evaluate the amount of vertical opening at the first point of contact and set the articulator.
   a. To set the articulator:
      - Loosen locks and incisal pin.
      - Squeeze into maximum intercuspation.
      - Set pin.
      - Return to centric relation.
   b. Set condylar inclination guided by:
      - Protrusive record
      - Clinical observations
      - Matching wear patterns
3. Evaluate anterior coupling. Work out edge-to-edge crossover details and the mandibular incisal plane. Then equilibrate posterior teeth as follows:
   a. Read receiving area.
   b. Warp offending cusp tip.
   c. Erase old incline mark.
4. Equilibrate anterior contacts:
   a. Level lower anteriors.
   b. Warp lower cuspids and bicuspids.
   c. Don't dig holes for CR stops.
   d. Maintain cuspid angle until posterior teeth are replaced.
   e. When appropriate, reduce vertical to return anterior stops.
5. Remove all balancing and protrusive interferences.
6. Analyze cuspid guidance.

7. Work out optimal anterior guidance.
8. Evaluate Curve of Wilson and refine anterior guidance.
9. Check the equilibration after establishing the maximum number of centric stops. Allow for freedom in centric, performing these excursions under pressure:
   - Inward as well outward
   - Crossover contacts
   Consider:
   - Habitual occlusion
   - Sleep positions
   - Tracking smoothness (Is there a trip or catch?)
10. Begin tap tapping, and refine centric stops to a halo and polish.

REFERENCES

Becker I.M., Tarantola, G., Zambrano, J., et al. (1999). Effect of a prefabricated anterior bite stop on electromyographic activity of masticatory muscles. *Journal of Prosthetic Dentistry*, Vol. 82, pp. 22–26.

Begg, P.R. (1954). Stone age man's dentition with reference to anatomically correct occlusion, the etiology of malocclusion, and a technique for its treatment. *American Journal of Orthodontics*, Vol. 40, pp. 298–312, 373–383, 517–531.

Berry, D.C., and Poole, D.F. (1976). Attrition: Possible mechanism of compensation. *Journal of Oral Rehabilitation*, Vol. 3, pp. 201–206.

Crothers, A.J. (1992). Tooth wear and facial morphology. *Journal of Dentistry*, Vol. 20, pp. 333–341.

Crothers, A.J., and Sandham, A. (1993). Vertical height differences in subjects with severe dental wear. *European Journal of Orthodontics*, Vol. 15, pp. 519–525.

Kaifu, Y., Kasai, K., Townsend, G., et al. (2008). Tooth to wear and the design of the human dentition: A perspective from evolutionary medicine. *Year Book of Physical Anthropology*, Vol. 46, pp. 47–61.

Karl, P.J., and Foley, T.F. (1999). The use of a deprogramming appliance to obtain centric relation records. *Angle Orthodontics* Vol. 69, pp. 117–123.

Lucia, V.O. (1964). A technique for recording centric relation. *Journal of Prosthetic Dentistry*, Vol. 14, pp. 492–505.

McKee, J.R. (1977). Comparing condylar position repeatability for standardized versus nonstandardized methods of achieving centric relation. *Journal Prosthetic Dentistry*, Vol. 77, pp. 280–284.

McKee, J.R. (2005). Comparing condylar positions achieved through bimanual manipulation to condylar positions achieved through masticatory muscle contraction against an anterior deprogrammer: A pilot study. *Journal Prosthetic Dentistry*, Vol. 94, pp. 389–393.

Murphy, T. (1959). Compensatory mechanism in facial height adjustment to functional tooth attrition. *Australian Dental Journal*, Vol. 4, pp. 312–323.

Riise, C. (1982). Rational performance of occlusal adjustment. *Journal of Prosthetic Dentistry*, Vol. 48, pp. 319–327.

Sicher, H. (1953). The biology of attrition. *Oral Surgery*, Vol. 6, pp. 406–412.

Solow, R.A. (1999). The anterior acrylic resin platform and centric relation verification: A clinical report. *Journal Prosthetic Dentistry*, Vol. 81, pp. 255–257.

Tarantola, G.J., Becker, I.M., and Gremillion, H. (1997). The reproducibility of centric relation: A clinical approach. *Journal of American Dental Association*, Vol. 128, pp. 1245–1251.

Whittaker, D.K., Molleson, T., Daniel, A.J., et al. (1985). Quantitative assessment of tooth wear, alveolar-crest height and continuing education. *Archives of Oral Biology*, Vol. 30, pp. 493–501.

Williamson, E.H., et al. (1980). Centric relation: A comparison of muscle-determined position and operator guidance. *American Journal of Orthodontics*, Vol. 77, pp. 133–145.

RECOMMENDED READING

Agar, J.R., and Weller, R.N. (1988). Occlusal adjustment for initial treatment and prevention of the cracked tooth syndrome. *Journal of Prosthetic Dentistry*, Vol. 60, pp. 145–147.

Au, A.R., and Klineberg, I.J. (1994). A new approach for accurate pre-planned occlusal adjustment. *Australian Dental Journal*, Vol. 39, pp. 11–14.

Belanger, G.K. (1992). The rationale and indications for equilibration in the primary dentition. *Quintessence International*, Vol. 23, pp. 169–174.

Christensen, G.J. (2005). The major part of dentistry you may be neglecting. *Journal of the American Dental Association*, Vol. 136, p. 4979.

Clark, G.T., and Adler, R.C. (1985). A critical evaluation of occlusal therapy: Occlusal adjustment procedures. *Journal of the American Dental Association*, Vol. 110, p. 743.

Hammad, I.A., Nassif, J.A., and Salameh, Z.A. (2005). Full-mouth rehabilitation following treatment of temporomandibular disorders and teeth-related signs and symptoms. *Journal of Craniomandibular Practice*, Vol. 23, pp. 289–296.

Kerstein, R.B. (1993). A comparison of traditional occlusal equilibration and immediate complete anterior guidance development. *Journal of Craniomandibular Practice*, Vol. 11, pp. 126–139.

Kerstein, R.B., and Farrell, S. (1990). Treatment of myofascial pain-dysfunction syndrome with occlusal equilibration. *Journal of Prosthetic Dentistry*, Vol. 63, pp. 695–700.

Kerstein, R.B., and Wright, N.R. (1991). Electromyographic and computer analyses of patients suffering from chronic myofascial pain-dysfunction syndrome: Before and after treatment with immediate complete anterior development. *Journal of Prosthetic Dentistry*, Vol. 66, pp. 677–686.

Kirveskari, P., et al. (1989) Effect of elimination of occlusal interferences on signs and symptoms of craniomandibular disorder in young adults. *Journal of Oral Rehabilitation*, Vol. 16, pp. 21–26.

Magne, P., and Belser, U.C. (2002). Rationalization of shape and related stress distribution in posterior teeth: A finite element study using nonlinear contact analysis. *International Journal of Periodontal Restorative Dentistry*, Vol. 22, pp. 425–433.

McHorris, W.H. (1985). Occlusal adjustment via selective cutting of natural teeth: Part I. *International Journal of Periodontal Restorative Dentistry*, Vol. 5, pp. 8–25.

Nassif, N.J. (2001). Perceived malocclusion and other teeth-associated signs and symptoms in temporomandibular disorders. *Compendium*, Vol. 22, pp. 577–584.

Okeson, J.P., Dickson, J.L., and Kemper, J.T. (1982). The influence of assisted mandibular movement on the incidence of nonworking contact. *Journal of Prosthetic Dentistry*, Vol. 48, pp. 174–177.

Ramfjord, S.P. (1961). Bruxism, a clinical and electromyographic study. *Journal of the American Dental Association*, Vol. 62, pp. 21–44.

Rosner, D. (1981). A chairside analysis of the feasibility of selective grinding. *Journal of Prosthetic Dentistry*, Vol. 54, pp. 30–36.

Schuyler, C.H. (1953). Factors in occlusion applicable to restorative dentistry. *Journal of Prosthetic Dentistry*, Vol. 3, p. 722.

Scotti, R., Villa, L., and Carossa, S. (1991). Clinical applicability of the radiographic method for determining the thickness of calcified crown tissues. *Journal of Prosthetic Dentistry*, Vol. 65, pp. 65–67.

Shillingburg, H.T., and Grace, C.S. (1973). Thickness of enamel and dentin. *Journal of South California Dental Association*, Vol. 41, pp. 33–52.

Tarantola, G.J., Becker, I.M., Gremillion, H., et al. (1998). The effectiveness of equilibration in the improvement of signs and symptoms in the stomatognathic system. *Journal of Periodontal Restorative Dentistry*, Vol. 18, pp. 595–603.

Williamson, E.H., and Simmons, M.D. (1978). Assessment of anterior tooth coupling and equilibration using a diagnostic mounting. *Quintessence International*, Vol. 10, pp. 61–66.

Winstanley, R.B. (1986). A retrospective analysis of the treatment of occlusal disharmony by selective grinding. *Journal of Oral Rehabilitation*, Vol. 13, pp. 169–181.

Wiskott, H.W.A., and Belser, U.C. (1995). A rationale for simplified occlusal design in restorative dentistry: Historical review and clinical guidelines. *Journal of Prosthetic Dentistry*, Vol. 73, pp. 69–83.

Ziebert, G.J., and Donegan, S.J. (1979). Tooth contacts and stability before and after occlusal adjustment. *Journal of Prosthetic Dentistry*, Vol. 42, pp. 276–281.

Dentist-Ceramist Communication, the Foundation of Successful Treatment

Matthew R. Roberts, CDT

To achieve a successful outcome when restoring a patient's dentition, we must first have a treatment plan based on the patient's needs, desires, and existing clinical condition. This treatment plan is the blueprint for successful completion of the patient's diagnosed treatment. It also designates the members of the treatment team and the specialist who will perform each procedure and in which order. The general dentist coordinates, directs, and choreographs the treatment procedures to idealize the outcome for the patient. This process requires detailed communication between the treating dentist and all members of the treatment team, allowing each to visualize the final outcome of the case and to understand what specifically is required of him or her to contribute to the final desired result.

Communication between the dentist and the ceramist in the dental laboratory is a critical but sometimes overlooked part of the overall treatment team communication. Visualization of the final desired result by the dental ceramist is critical to the successful completion of the restorative prosthesis. The protocol for this communication and the tools available to complete it have evolved rapidly over the last ten years. The integration of digital photography, e-mail communication, and easy video conferencing with Skype or iChat has greatly enhanced the communication process. There is still, however, the need for a basic blueprint that defines, in detail, the restorative plan for each patient and organizes this into a plan of action. The laboratory prescription fills this need and is the foundation upon which communication essential to the case is built.

Comprehensive Occlusal Concepts in Clinical Practice, by Irwin M. Becker
© 2011 Blackwell Publishing Ltd.

The laboratory prescription answers these basic questions:

- Which teeth are to be restored utilizing which restorative materials?
- What future phases of treatment are to be completed that may affect the current phase of treatment?
- When is the case to be delivered?
- What shade is desired?
- How much translucency?
- How much surface morphology?
- What tooth length?
- Is vertical dimension being opened?
- Is the bite registration based on centric relation or maximum intercuspation?

It is also helpful for the ceramist to understand the patient's goals and preferences before fabricating the restorations. To accomplish this communication, a *comprehensive* lab prescription is used (fig. 11.1).

Esthetic and reconstructive aspects of comprehensive, multiunit anterior cases require further, specialized communication to allow the ceramist to visualize and create an outcome that accomplishes the treatment goals and is pleasing esthetically to the patient. After review of the information in the lab prescription, which lays out the basics, communication of facial orientation of the dentition is necessary for esthetic success. All of the things that are sent to the lab—bite registrations, models of provisional restorations, and master casts of the prepared teeth, need to be related to the patient's facial features to understand how the dental component relates to the rest of the patient's facial features.

The clinician needs to tell the ceramist where to put the teeth by doing the following:

- defining the vertical midline,
- identifying the horizontal plane,
- locating the facial-lingual location of the maxillary incisal edge,
- quantifying the length of the teeth,
- establishing the relationship of mandibular teeth to maxillary teeth,
- communicating the amount of tooth display (and gingival display) at a high smile,
- communicating the shape of the teeth desired by the patient,
- communicating the tooth shade desired by the patient,
- communicating the arrangement of the teeth desired by the patient, and
- defining the color of the underlying dentition if all-ceramic restorations or porcelain margins on PFM restorations are to be used.

Traditional tools such as a facebow are still very valuable; they transfer the relationship of the teeth to the temporomandibular joint, along with the

CMR Dental Lab

Submit by Email

Print Form

Matt Roberts 185 S. Capital Ave. Idaho Falls, ID 83402 208-523-3401 Fax 208-523-0937

Date _____   Due Date _____

Doctor _____   Telephone Number _____

Address _____

Name of Patient _____   Gender _____   Age _____

Items Included with Case

- ○ Master Impression
- ○ Opposing impression or model
- ○ Stick bite
- ○ Bite registration

- ○ Diagnostic wax-up
- ○ Model or impression of provisionals
- ○ Pre-operative models
- ○ Photos (Qty.__) Slides (Qty.__)

- ○ Face bow transfer jig
- ○ Other _____
  _____

○	○	○	○	○	○	○	○	○	○	○	○	○	○	○	○
1	2	3	4	5	6	7	8	9	10	11	12	13	14	15	16
32	31	30	29	28	27	26	25	24	23	22	21	20	19	18	17
○	○	○	○	○	○	○	○	○	○	○	○	○	○	○	○

Goals of Final Case

Type of Restoration Desired

- ○ Feldspathic -teeth #s _____
- ○ Empress Esthetic -teeth #s _____
- ○ Emax -Lithium Disilicate-teeth #s _____
- ○ Emax -Pressed over Zirconia-teeth #s _____

- ○ PFG -teeth #s _____
- ○ Resin -teeth #s _____
- ○ Other -teeth #s _____

Vertical Dimension   ○ Open Bite

Vertical measurement_____ mm   CEJ tooth #_____ to CEJ tooth #_____

Fig. 11.1. Comprehensive lab prescription. Courtesy of Matt Roberts and CMR Dental Lab.

resultant arc of excursive movements and the angle of the occlusal plane from anterior to posterior. Unfortunately, the complexity of using an ear bow system with a large amount of hardware with multiple locking points, combined with facial asymmetries often seen in patients, makes this system inferior for transferring the absolute vertical and horizontal plane. Discrepancies of two degrees of canting of the vertical midline are easily distinguishable visually by patients, and a more accurate system is needed to achieve accuracy.

Length

Centrals (tooth # ___) ___ mm Laterals (tooth # ___) ___ mm less than centrals Canine (tooth # ___) ___ mm

Any special length instructions ___

Shape

- Smile guide design # ___
- Smile catalog design ___
- Other ___
- Match photographs included ___
- Match contralateral ___

Shade of Preparation

Stump shade teeth #s ___ ST ___ Stump shade teeth #s ___ ST ___

Stump shade teeth #s ___ ST ___ Stump shade teeth #s ___ ST ___

Shade

Body Shade ___ Gingival shade ___ Incisal shade ___ Occlusal staining ___

Incisal Translucency

- Minimal (0.5mm)
- Moderate (1.0mm)
- Maximum (1.5mm)

Shade of Incisal Translucency

- Clear
- Smoke
- Frosted
- Amber

Surface Texture

- High
- Medium
- Light
- Smooth (no surface texture)

Surface Finish

- High glaze
- Polished gloss
- Satin finish
- Low gloss

Ingot Choice for Empress Esthetic (Optional)

- 01
- TC1
- OC1
- 02
- TC0
- 03
- Other

Degree of Opacity (Feldspathic)

- None
- Minimal (25%)
- Medium (50%)
- Maximum (100%)

- Provide reduction coping if necessary to improve aesthetics, reduce opposing or call and ask to re-prep

Miscellaneous Information

Doctor's Signature ___ License # ___

A Charge of 1.75% per month (21% APR) will be applied to all past due accounts. In event of collection action, debtor agrees to pay all collection costs, including attorney fees

Fig. 11.1. *Continued*

Stone casts of the provisional models, along with proper digital photography of the provisional restorations, are the most valuable tools we have today. A set of communication digital photographs are used to help a dental technician visualize how the patient's teeth relate to their facial features (see figs. 11.2–11.5). The stone cast of the provisional restorations is used to create a silicone mold of the provisional restorations, which is then seated over the prepared tooth model; wax is injected to accurately

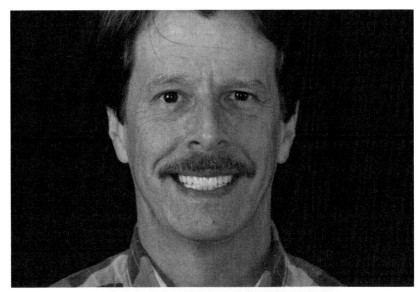

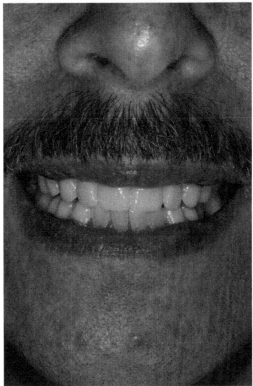

Figs. 11.2–11.5. Photos of provisional restorations, when combined with a stone cast of the provisionals, provide the blueprint for the ceramist to follow when fabricating the final case. The full face photo shows vertical midline and overall orientation of the smile to facial features, while the closer view provides more detail about the appearance of individual teeth. The lateral views show how protrusive or retrusive the provisionals are as well as the location of the incisal edge relative to the wet/dry line of the lip. Courtesy of Dr. Tom Trinkner.

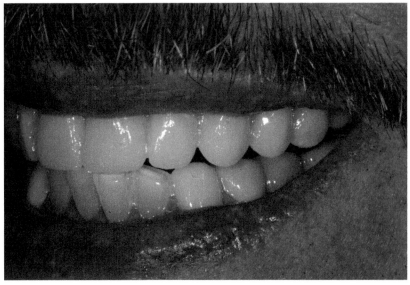

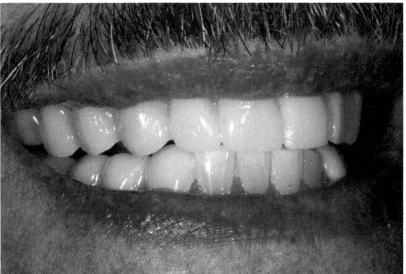

Figs. 11.2–11.5. *Continued*

replicate the provisionals. This not only transfers the esthetic features and orientation of the provisional restorations, it also transfers the lingual contours and the functional envelope. The ceramist can now start to look at a full series of photographs and make any changes that would visually improve the case, safe with the knowledge that he or she is starting from a known position. This takes the guesswork out of the communication and keeps all changes relevant to the patient's clinical situation.

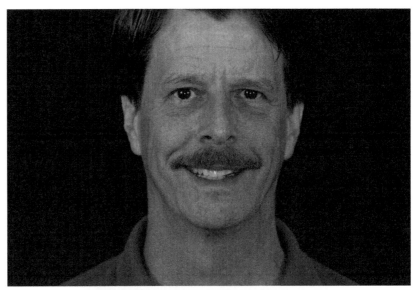

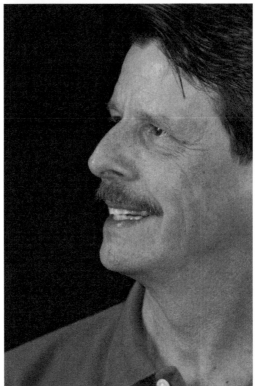

Figs. 11.6–11.13. Series of preoperative digital photographs are used while completing the diagnostic phase of treatment planning. Courtesy of Dr. Tom Trinkner.

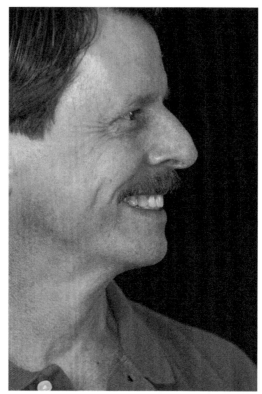

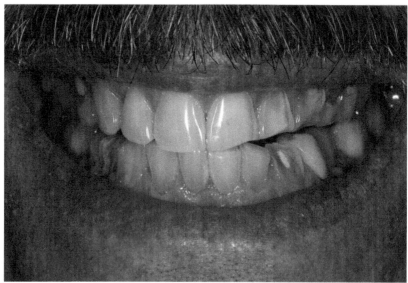

Figs. 11.6–11.13. *Continued*

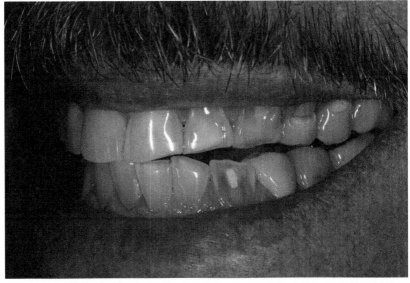

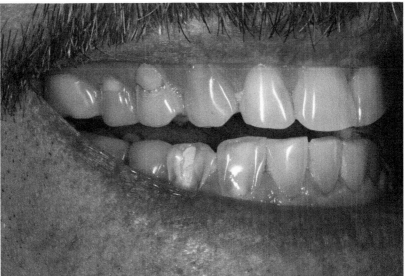

Figs. 11.6–11.13. *Continued*

Another very effective way of transferring horizontal (and by 90-degree interpretation, vertical) is through the use of a stick bite (fig. 11.14). This is a straight plastic stick that is incorporated into a rigid, fast-setting bite-registration material that is applied to the incisal edge of the mandibular anterior teeth. The stick is positioned to the facial of the lower teeth and close to the incisal edge of the maxillary central incisors. The stick is oriented in the horizontal plane while the patient stands, directly facing the

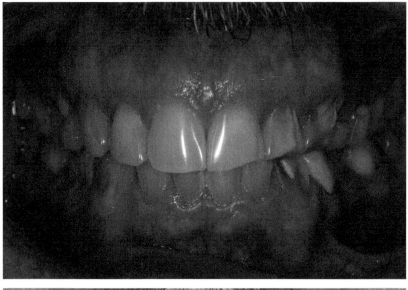

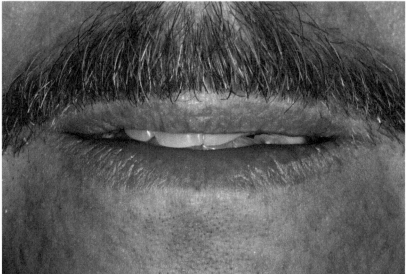

Figs. 11.6–11.13. *Continued*

dentist. The patient is instructed not to fully close, preventing the lower incisors from touching the lingual of the uppers and shearing off the lingual component of the bite. After the bite material sets, a photograph is taken to ensure the stick is in a level relationship to facial features. In the laboratory, the stick bite is placed on the lower anterior teeth and the wax-up of the upper arch is gently closed to the stick to evaluate the vertical midline and the horizontal plane of the case. The use of this technique greatly reduces the number of cases that appear canted on delivery.

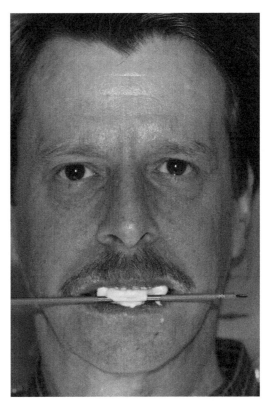

Fig. 11.14. The stick bite photograph is taken to be sure the stick is level with the interpupillary line and perpendicular to the long axis of the face. Courtesy of Dr. Tom Trinkner.

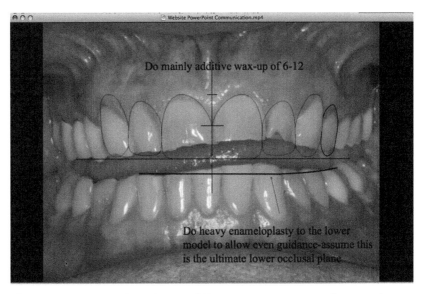

Figs. 11.15–11.17. PowerPoint and Keynote presentations can be created to act as a laboratory prescription. The ability to combine photos and text with lines and shaded areas make a powerful communication tool between the dentist and the restorative team. Courtesy of Dr. Jim Fondriest.

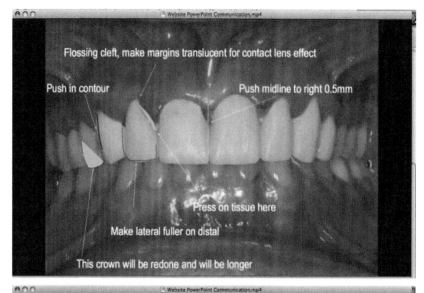

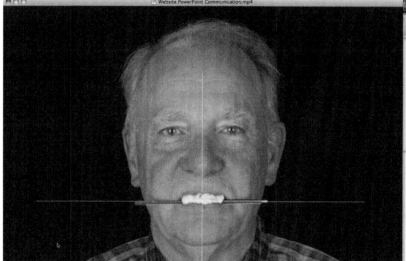

Figs. 11.15–11.17. *Continued*

Communication of color is heavily dependent on good photography. A shade tab is placed in the view of the camera, oriented the same way as the patient's teeth, and multiple photos are taken from various angles, thus moving the flash reflections to different parts of the tooth and allowing the ceramist to see internal details of the tooth structure in all areas (see figs. 11.18–11.22). Underexposed and overexposed photos can be very misleading; the practitioner should look at the photos while the patient is still there

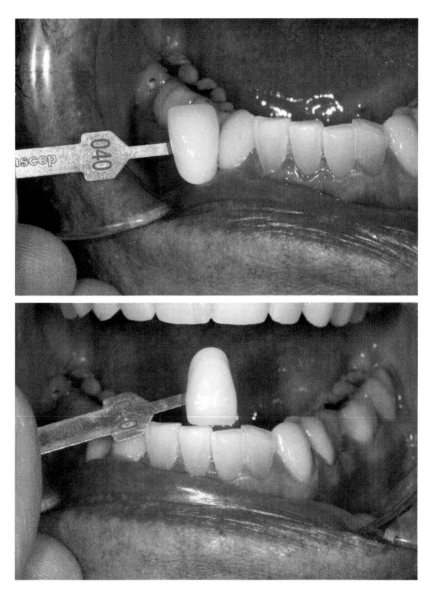

Figs. 11.18–11.22. Photographs showing the color of the underlying prepared teeth; this allows the ceramist to choose the appropriate ingot. These also demonstrate the selection of final desired shades. Courtesy of Dr. Tom Trinkner.

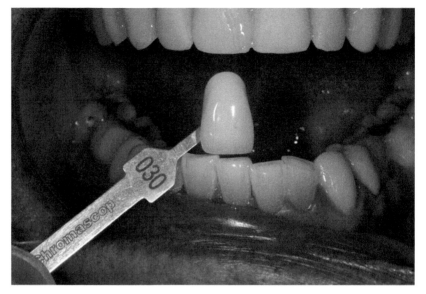

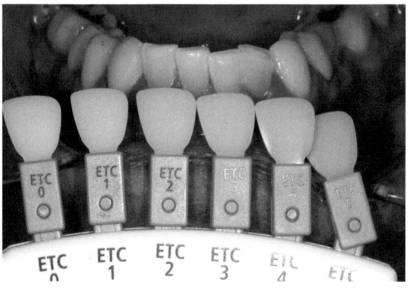

Figs. 11.18–11.22. *Continued*

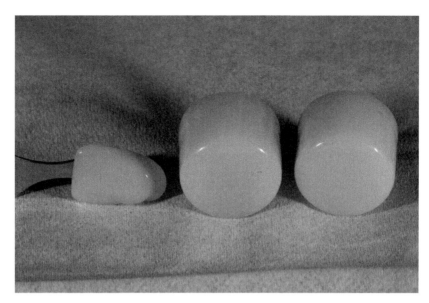

Figs. 11.18–11.22. *Continued*

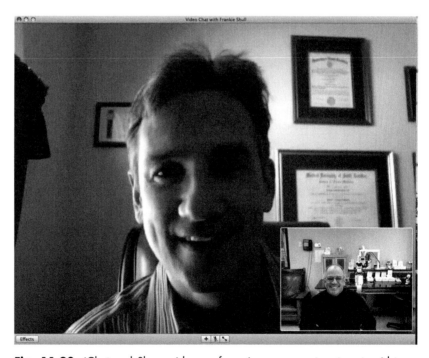

Fig. 11.23. iChat and Skype video conferencing are easy to set up to aid team communication. In the photo shown, Dr. Frankie Shull and Matt Roberts are discussing a case, passing photos back and forth and viewing Keynote presentations as though they are sitting in the same room, when actually, Frankie is in South Carolina and Matt is in Idaho. If team members are across town or across the country, this is a very effective means of communication.

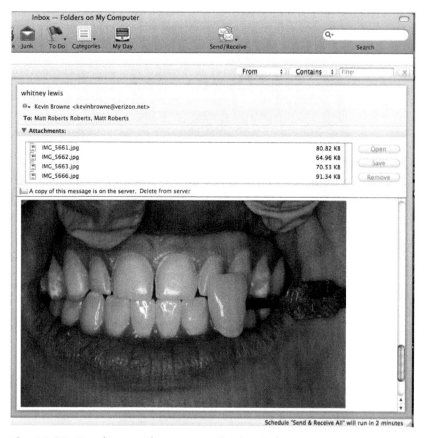

Fig. 11.24. E-mail is a quick way to transfer digital photos to team members. Any time a question comes up about a case in the laboratory, a photo showing the situation is e-mailed to the treating dentist. This can be followed with a phone call or an iChat session.

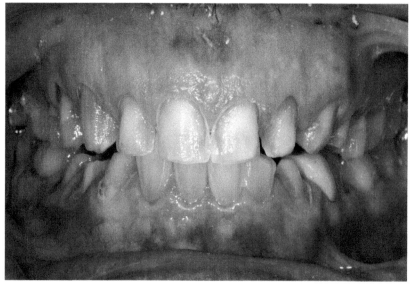

Figs. 11.25–11.27. A series of photographs demonstrating tooth preparations and requisite clearances and dimensions. Courtesy of Dr. Tom Trinkner.

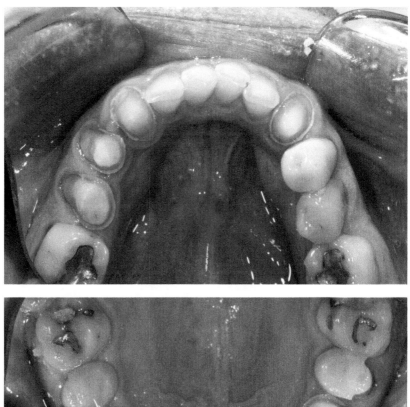

Figs. 11.25–11.27. *Continued*

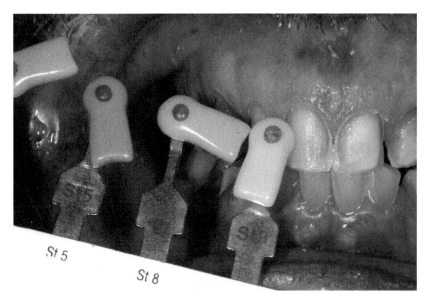

Fig. 11.28. Another photograph showing the color of the underlying prepared teeth, which aids the ceramist in choosing the appropriate ingot. Courtesy of Dr. Tom Trinkner.

and be sure that what is seen in the photo is representative of what is observed clinically. A hand-drawn shade map can be of value if the dentist has extensive knowledge of ceramic layering, but photos should also be included.

THE LAB COMMUNICATION PROTOCOL SUMMARIZED

- Perform esthetic composite mock-up (free hand).
- Provide facebow, CR records, and esthetic bite stick records.
- Provide comprehensive photographic documentation.
- Provide diagnostic wax-up.
- Provide composite application of wax-up.
- Communicate prep design.
- Prep and provisionalize from wax-up.
- Refine and reevaluate provisionals.
- Make comprehensive models and cross-mounting records.

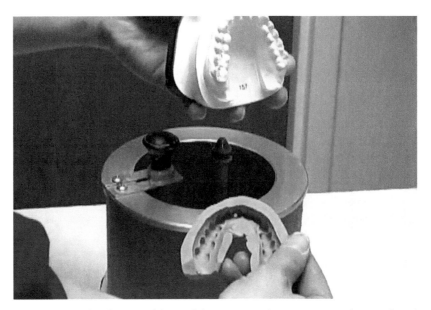

Fig. 11.29. The shape and form of the provisional restoration can be transferred to the definitive restorations via wax injection. A silicone matrix of the provisional is prepared with a small hole drilled in the incisor. This matrix is placed on the prepared tooth model and wax is injected through the incisal hole.

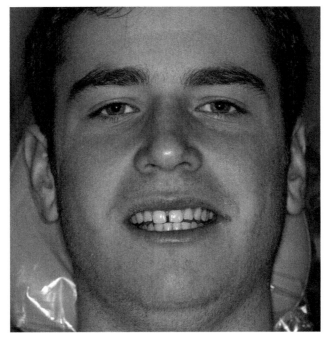

Figs. 11.30–11.35. A diastema closure case treated with very thin lithium disilicate veneers. Embrasure form is critical to prevent the final restorations from appearing too wide when closing spaces. Courtesy of Dr. Kevin Browne.

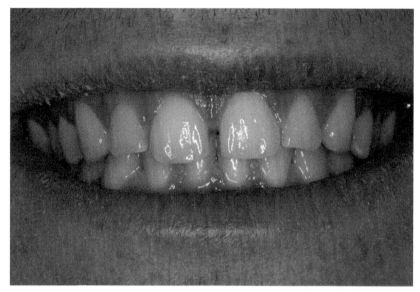

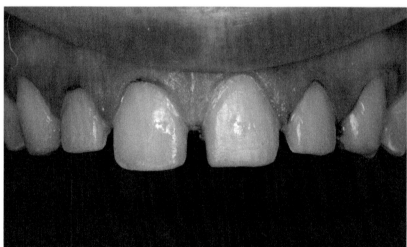

Figs. 11.30–11.35. *Continued*

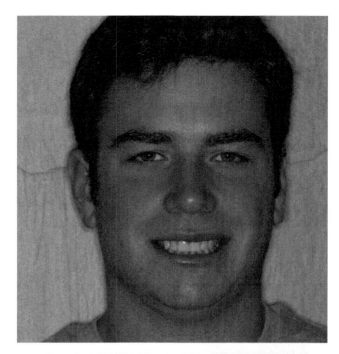

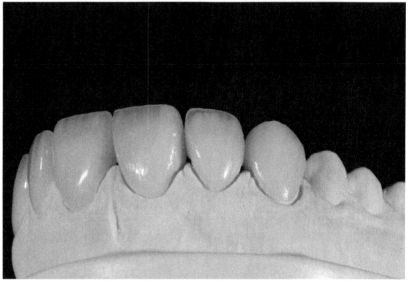

Figs. 11.30–11.35. *Continued*

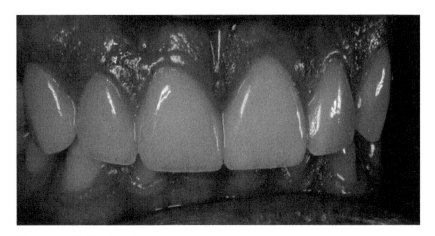

Figs. 11.30–11.35. *Continued*

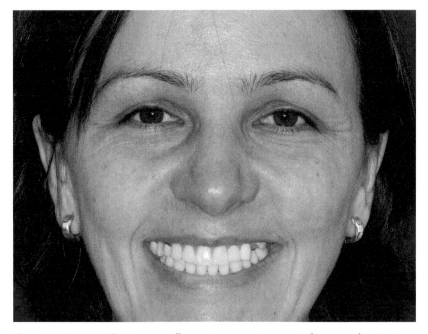

Figs. 11.36–11.39. Empress all-ceramic restorations revitalize a smile. Courtesy of Dr. Jim Fondriest.

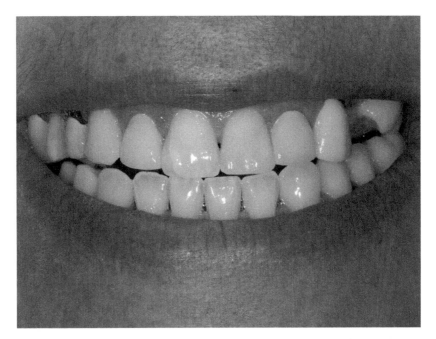

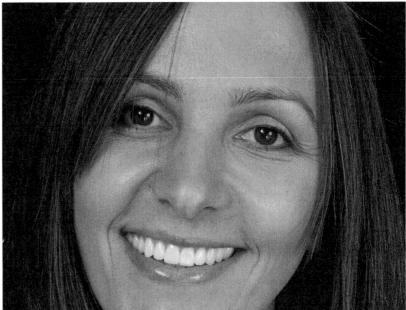

Figs. 11.36–11.39. *Continued*

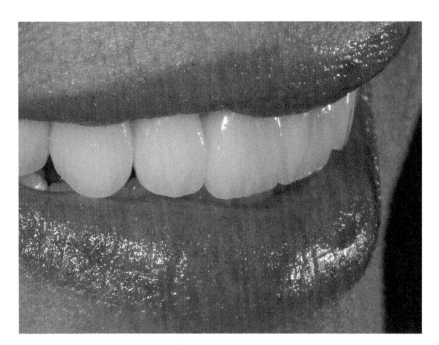

Figs. 11.36–11.39. *Continued*

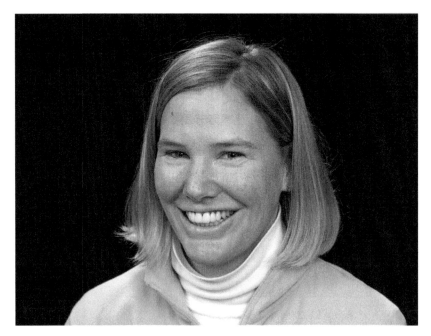

Figs. 11.40–11.44. Previous restorations left a lot to be desired from an esthetic and functional standpoint. By changing contour and material, there is potential to make vast improvement in overall appearance and function of a patient's smile. Courtesy of Dr Jim Fondriest.

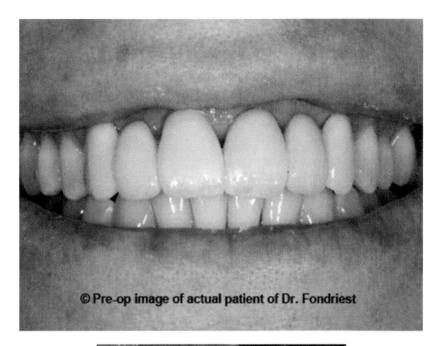

© Pre-op image of actual patient of Dr. Fondriest

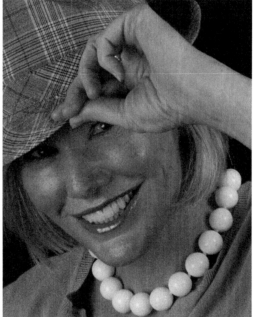

Figs. 11.40–11.44. *Continued*

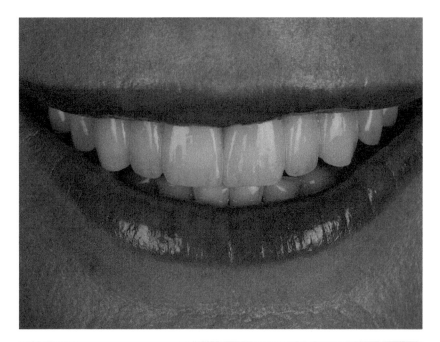

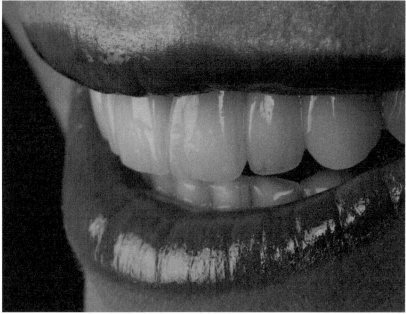

Figs. 11.40–11.44. *Continued*

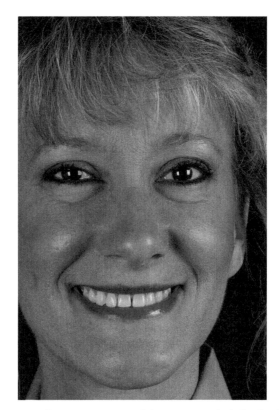

Fig. 11.45. Comprehensive treatment of this patient included orthodontics to position teeth prior to veneering with high-translucency lithium disilicate restorations. By following the diagnostic and communication steps in this chapter, the final result was achieved while retaining most of the patient's existing tooth structure. Final restorative thickness of the anterior teeth averaged 0.2–0.3 mm in this case. Courtesy of Dr. Franklin Shull.

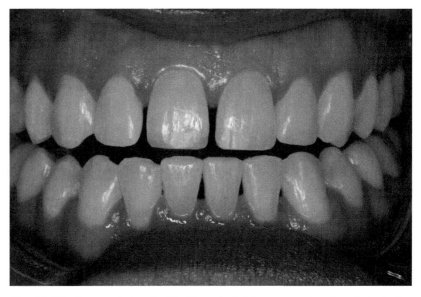

Fig. 11.46. Retracted view (1:2) with teeth slightly separated to show incisal edge discrepancies and tooth position in the arch. Courtesy of Dr. Franklin Shull.

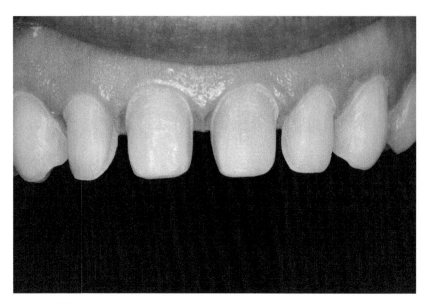

Fig. 11.47. Conservative veneer preparations to preserve enamel. Courtesy of Dr. Franklin Shull.

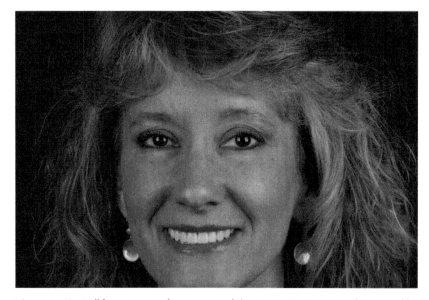

Fig. 11.48. Full-face image of a more confident patient. Courtesy of Dr. Franklin Shull.

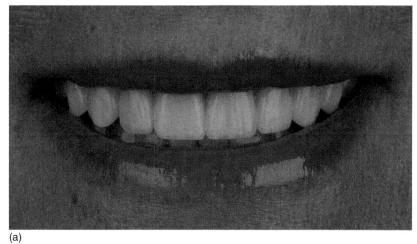

(a)

(b)

Fig. 11.49. a. Smile post-delivery. b. Close-up lateral view of post-delivery smile. Courtesy of Dr. Franklin Shull.

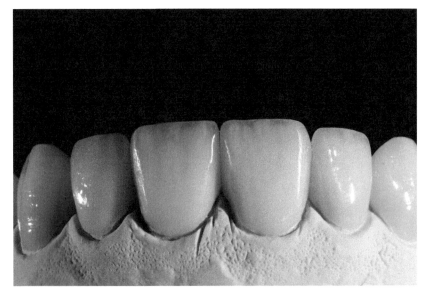

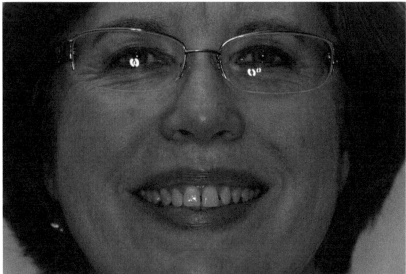

Figs. 11.50–11.59. This patient wanted improvement in the arrangement of her teeth without the appearance of having veneers. Spaces were filled and natural tooth color was allowed to show through the restorations in a very controlled way with very little removal of the patient's tooth structure. A high-translucency lithium disilicate was used as a restorative material. Courtesy of Dr. J. A. Reynolds.

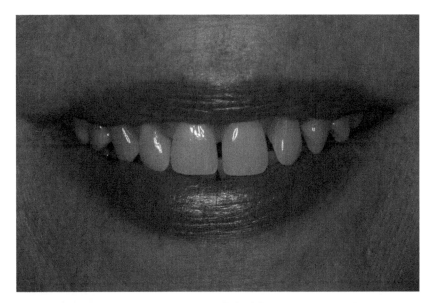

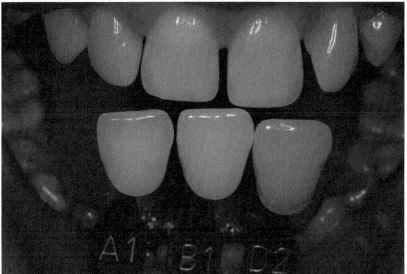

Figs. 11.50–11.59. *Continued*

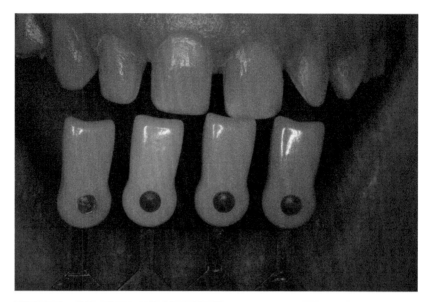

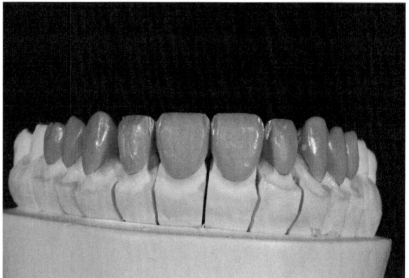

Figs. 11.50–11.59. *Continued*

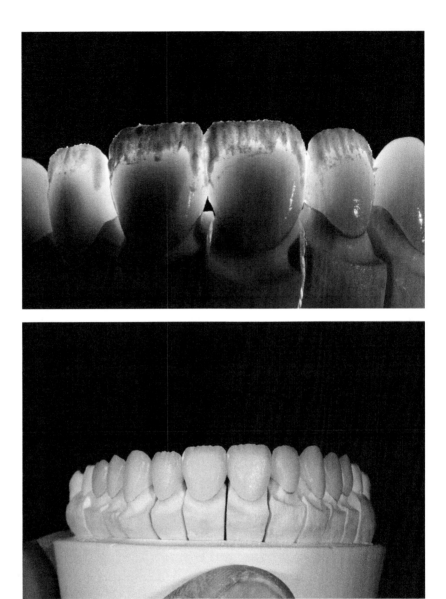

Figs. 11.50–11.59. *Continued*

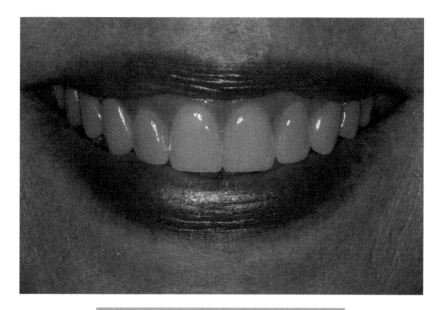

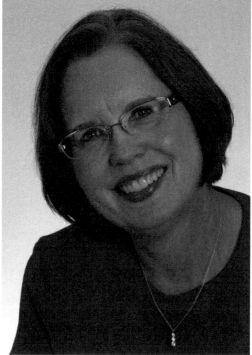

Figs. 11.50–11.59. *Continued*

Index

Comprehensive Occlusal Concepts in Clinical Practice, by Irwin M. Becker
© 2011 Blackwell Publishing Ltd.

Printed and bound by CPI Group (UK) Ltd, Croydon, CR0 4YY

16/04/2025

14658464-0001